ECONOMICS
for HEALTHCARE
MANAGERS

ECONOMICS for HEALTHCARE MANAGERS

ROBERT H. LEE

Health Administration Press, Chicago, Illinois
AUPHA Press, Washington, D.C.

AUPHA
HAP

04 03 02 01 00   5 4 3 2 1

The paper used in this publication meets the minimum requirements of American National Standard for Information Sciences—Permanence of Paper for Printed Library Materials, ANSW Z39.48–1984.

Library of Congress Cataloging-in-Publication Data

Lee, Robert H., 1948–
    Economics for healthcare managers / Robert H. Lee
        p. cm.
    Includes bibliographical references and index.
    ISBN 1-56793-130-8 (alk. paper)
    1. Health services administration—Economic aspects.   2. Medical economics.
3. Managerial economics.   I. Title.

    RA427 .L44 2000
    362.1'068'1—dc21

                                                                    00-039699

Health Administration Press
A division of the Foundation of the
    American College of Healthcare Executives
1 North Franklin Street, Suite 1700
Chicago, IL 60606–3491
(312) 424–2800

Association of University Programs
    in Health Administration
1911 North Fort Meyer Drive
Suite 503
Arlington, VA 22209
(703) 524–5500

CONTENTS

WHY HEALTH ECONOMICS?

Key Concepts

- Economics helps managers focus on key issues.
- Economics helps managers understand goal-oriented decision making.
- Economics helps managers understand strategic decision making.
- Economics gives managers a framework for understanding costs.
- Economics gives managers a framework for understanding market demand.
- Economics gives managers a framework for assessing profitability.

1.1 Why Health Economics?

Why should working healthcare managers study economics? This simple question is really two questions: Why is economics valuable for managers? What special challenges do healthcare managers face? These questions motivate this book.

Why is economics valuable for managers? In this chapter, we will briefly touch on the following six reasons why economics is valuable to highlight the themes that we will develop more fully in later chapters:

1. *Economics helps managers focus on key issues.* Economics helps managers to wade through the deluge of information that they confront and to identify the data that they really need.
2. *Economics outlines strategies for realizing goals given the available resources.* We will explore carefully the implications of economics on rational decision making.
3. *Economics gives managers ground rules for decision making when their rivals are not only competing against them, but watching what they do.* Later, we will explore how an understanding of economics can aid in strategic planning and decision making.
4. *Economics gives managers a framework for making sense of costs.* A crucial part of a manager's job is the need to understand how to manage costs.
5. *Economics provides an explicit framework for thinking about how much consumers value goods and services.* Other disciplines may offer more insight into what motivates consumers, but economics gives managers a firm understanding of what consumers value.
6. *More than anything, economics sensitizes managers to fundamental ideas that affect the operations of every organization.* Effective management must begin with the recognition that consumers are sensitive to price

differences, that organizations compete to advance the interests of their stakeholders, and that success comes from giving consumers value.

1.2 Economics as a Map for Decision Making

Economics provides a map for decision making. Maps do two things: They highlight key features and suppress unimportant features. If you drive from Des Moines, Iowa to Dallas, Texas, you need to know how the major highways connect. You do not need to know the name and location of each street in each town you pass through along the way. Of course, what is important and what is unimportant depends on the task at hand. If you drive from Burch Street and Ridgeview Road in Olathe, Kansas to the Truman homestead in Independence, Missouri, a map that describes only the interstate highway system will be of limited value to you. You need to know which map is the right tool for your particular situation.

Using a map takes both knowledge and skill. You must know what information you need, or else you may choose the wrong map and be swamped in extraneous data or be lost without key facts. But simply having the right map is no guarantee that you can use it. You must practice using maps to learn to use one quickly and effectively. In this sense as well, economics serves as a map for decision making.

Like a map, economics highlights some issues and suppresses others. For example, economics tells managers to focus on incremental costs, which makes understanding and managing costs much simpler. At the same time, however, economics has little or nothing to say about the health belief systems that motivate consumer behavior. If you are seeking to make therapeutic regimens easier to adhere to by making them more consistent with consumers' belief systems, economics is not a very helpful map. If, on the other hand, you want to decide whether it will be feasible to set up an urgent care clinic, economics helps you focus on how that will change revenues and costs. This sort of simplification can be very helpful to managers who are deluged with information.

Economics also gives managers a framework for understanding rational decision making. Rational decision making entails making choices that further one's goals given the available resources. Whether those goals include maximizing profits, securing the health of the indigent, or other objectives, the framework is much the same. It entails looking at both benefits and costs to realize the largest net benefit. (We will explore this question somewhat further in Section 1.5.)

Obviously, this framework for rational decision making requires a clear understanding of costs and benefits. Economics provides the basis for this understanding. Managers must understand costs and be able to explain them to others. Confusion about costs is common, so confused decision making is also common. Confusion about benefits is, if anything, more widespread than confusion about costs. As a result, management decisions in healthcare often leave much to be desired.

The enthusiasm of economists for "perfectly competitive markets" (which are, for the most part, mythical social structures) obscures the contribution of economics for managers who are competing in real-world markets. In reality, economics offers concrete guidance about pricing, contracting, and other quandaries that managers face in their "imperfect" worlds. Economics also offers a framework for evaluating the sorts of strategic choices that many managers must make. Many healthcare organizations compete with a small number of rivals. As a result, good decisions must take into account the actions of the competition. Will being the first to enter a market give your organization an advantage or will it give your rivals a low-cost way of observing what works and what does not? Will buying primary care practices bring you increased market share or "buyer's remorse"? A knowledge of economics will not make these choices easy, but it can give managers a plan for sorting through the issues.

Hospitals Learn About Incentives and Buyer's Remorse

In recent years, many hospitals have acquired physician practices. Nearly all of those hospitals are losing money on what were once profitable practices. Economics gives two important insights into the unhappiness of hospitals with their purchases.

First, most practice purchases were knee-jerk responses to what competitors were doing, rather than carefully considered business plans. Enamored by the fact that physicians typically generate large inpatient revenues for each dollar of outpatient revenue that they generate, hospitals typically did not ask two key questions, "How will buying these practices change the amount of inpatient revenues that physicians will bring us?" and "Why are physicians willing to sell?" We still do not know the answer to the first question. The answer to the second question is quite simple—hospitals overpaid. Hospitals started buying just as practice valuations began dropping as a result of the growth of managed care and the increasing competition for patients.

Second, hospitals ignored incentives. Most hospitals converted from compensation based on billings to salaries after they acquired practices, which was a significant mistake. Economics reminds us that incentives matter. For physicians whose earnings depend on billings, the marginal patient, the patient squeezed in at the end of the day, or the patient booked in anticipation that someone will cancel, is highly profitable. For physicians whose earnings depend on salaries, in contrast, the marginal patient is financially unrewarding. Not surprisingly, Richard Haugh reports that physicians in independent practice produced 38 percent more procedures than those in practices owned by hospitals (1998). In recent years, hospitals have been rewriting compensation contracts, returning to incentive-based pay. Hospitals that have done so have seen productivity turn around, once again confirming economists' emphasis on incentives.

1.3 Special challenges for healthcare managers

What special challenges do healthcare managers face? Five issues challenge health-care managers more than other managers:

1. the central roles of risk and uncertainty;
2. insurance;
3. information asymmetries;
4. not-for-profit organizations; and
5. the rapid and confusing pace of technical and institutional change.

We will look at each of these in turn.

1.3.1 Risk and Uncertainty

Risk and uncertainty are defining features of healthcare markets and healthcare organizations. Both the incidence of illness and the effectiveness of medical care should be described in terms of probabilities. For example, the correct therapy, done correctly, usually carries a risk of failure. Some proportion of patients will experience harmful side effects and some proportion of patients will not benefit. As a result, cost management and quality management present managers with difficult challenges. Has a provider with bad outcomes had the bad luck to treat an extremely sick panel of patients, the bad luck to encounter a panel of patients for whom standard therapies are ineffective, the bad luck to have been let down by his or her colleagues, or the bad luck to be incompetent, sloppy, or lazy? It can be hard to tell.

1.3.2 Insurance

Because risk and uncertainty are of such great consequence in healthcare, most consumers have medical insurance. As a result, healthcare organizations must contend with the management problems that insurance presents. To begin with, insurance creates confusion about who the customer is. To be sure, the consumer receives the care, but insurance plans often pay most of the bill. Moreover, con-fusion often exists about who the insurer's customer is. Most people with private medical insurance get coverage through their employer (in large part because the tax system makes doing so inexpensive). Although economists generally agree that employees ultimately pay for insurance via wage reductions, employees often do not know the full cost of their insurance alternatives (and, unless they are changing jobs, have limited interest in finding out). This lack of knowledge further isolates consumers from the true cost of their care and makes them less eager to balance the cost of the care against its value.

In addition, insurance makes even simple transactions complex. Most insurance-related transactions involve at least three parties (the patient, the insurer, and the provider), and many involve more. Because most providers deal with a wide array of insurance plans, they face, as a result, a blizzard of disparate claim forms and payment systems. Increasing numbers of insurance plans have negotiated individual payment systems and rates, so many healthcare providers look wistfully at industries that get their revenues by simply billing clients.

This complexity, moreover, expands the possibilities for both mistakes and fraud to occur. No student of history will be surprised to learn that both are fairly common in transactions that involve health insurance. Yet this bewildering array of insurance plans does not save providers from dependence on a few plans (a circumstance that most managers seek to avoid). For example, most hospitals get at least a third of their revenue from Medicare. As a result, changes in Medicare regulations or payment methods can profoundly alter the prospects of a healthcare organization. Practically overnight, changes in reimbursement may transform a market from one in which everyone makes a profit to one in which only the strongest, best-led, and best-positioned can survive.

1.3.3 Information Asymmetries

Along with the seemingly endless issues concerning insurance, healthcare managers face unique challenges relating to information management. Information asymmetries are common in healthcare markets and they can create a number of problems. An information asymmetry occurs when one party in a transaction has more information than the other party. The party with less information runs the risk of being taken advantage of or, because of fears of being taken advantage of, not making a transaction that would be beneficial for him or her. For example, physicians and other healthcare providers usually understand patients' medical options better than the patients do. As a result, patients may accept recommendations for therapies that are not cost-effective or, recognizing their vulnerability to self-serving advice, may resist recommendations that are highly beneficial.

From the perspective of healthcare managers, asymmetric information means that physicians have a great deal of autonomy in recommending therapies. Because physicians' recommendations largely define the operations of insurance plans, hospitals, and group practices, managers must ensure that physicians do not have incentives to take advantage of their superior information. Information asymmetries also create an environment in which patients are likely to be able to make better forecasts of their healthcare use than insurers. Patients know whether they want to start a family, whether they seek medical attention whenever they feel ill, or whether they have symptoms that may mean they have an ulcer. As a result, health plans are vulnerable to adverse selection, or differential enrollment of high-cost customers.

1.3.4 Not-for-Profit Organizations

Not-for-profit organizations are common in healthcare. This is not a bad thing. Most not-for-profit organizations have worthy goals that their managers take seriously. But even not-for-profit organizations with lofty aspirations create some unique problems for healthcare managers. One problem arises because not-for-profit organizations usually have multiple stakeholders. When multiple stakeholders exist, multiple goals exist as well. When organizations have multiple goals, they become much more difficult to manage and the performance of managers becomes more difficult to assess. The potential for managers to put their own needs before their stakeholders' needs exists in all organizations, but is likely to be greater in not-for-profit organizations because there is no simple "bottom line." In addition, not-for-profit organizations may be more challenging to run well because they operate amid a web of regulations that are designed to prevent them from being used as tax avoidance schemes. These regulations make it difficult to set up incentive-based compensation systems for managers, employees, and contractors (the most important of whom are physicians). It is also difficult to convert the resources of not-for-profit organizations to other uses when programs are cut or cancelled. Because of these special challenges, managers of not-for-profit organizations can always claim that substandard performance reflects their more complex environment.

1.3.5 The Confusing Course of Change

This fifth challenge makes the others pale in comparison. The healthcare system is in a state of turmoil. Virtually every part of the healthcare sector is at work reinventing itself—technology, research, payment systems, and even the individual caregiving institutions themselves. Worse still, no one really knows where the healthcare system is headed. The job of leading an organization is quite difficult if you do not know where you are going. Because change is such a pervasive challenge facing healthcare managers today, let's examine it in greater detail.

1.4 Turmoil in the U.S. Healthcare System

Why is the healthcare system of the United States in such turmoil? One explanation is common to all the developed world: rapid technical change. The pace of medical research and development is breathtaking, and the public's desire for better therapies is manifest. The challenge of meeting this demand forces healthcare managers to lead their organizations into unmapped territory nearly every day. If this were not enough, the imperative to embrace these changes, most of which were designed to make the delivery of healthcare services more efficient and less costly, co-exists with (and contributed to the creation of) a significant surplus of physicians and hospital beds. Advances in technology, changes in insurance, and the continuation of long-standing policies that were designed to expand the capacity of the healthcare system have combined to create a system with significant *excess* capacity. Neither policy makers nor healthcare managers are prepared to lead the system through an era of downsizing.

1.4.1 The Pressure to Reduce Costs

The economics of high healthcare costs are far simpler than the political implications of high healthcare costs on a national level. To reduce costs, healthcare providers must reallocate resources from low-productivity uses to high-productivity uses, increase productivity wherever feasible, and reduce prices paid to suppliers and sectors where excess supply exists. This said, managers must recognize that cutting costs is very difficult at the national political level. Reallocating resources and increasing productivity will cost some people their jobs. Reducing prices will lower incomes for some people. These are difficult steps for any government to permit (and even more difficult for a government to take directly), and many of those who will be affected (physicians, nurses, or hospital employees) are politically well organized. The political problem is compounded because the real cost of healthcare is so fragmented. Most Americans see only a fraction of the actual cost of their healthcare. A typical American pays his or her share of healthcare costs through a mixture of direct payments for care; payroll deductions for insurance premiums; lower wages; higher prices for goods and services; and federal, state, and local taxes. Because of all of these "hidden" costs, it is no surprise that most Americans cannot track actual healthcare costs. The exceptions, notably the employers who write checks for the entire cost of insurance policies and the trustees of the Medicare system, better understand the need to reduce costs. Because so few Americans recognize how much their healthcare actually costs, changes in the complex system of public regulations and subsidies will be slow at best.

Why is the pressure to reduce healthcare costs so strong?

The answer is quite simple. The United States spends far more on healthcare than other wealthy industrial countries, but fares worse on health indicators than most of them (Anderson 1997). Spending per person is 67 percent higher than spending in Germany and 85 percent higher than spending in Canada, the two countries with the next highest levels of spending. Differences this large should be reflected in the outcomes of care.

	Share of GDP spent on health[a]		Spending per person[b]	
	1990	1996	1990	1996
Canada	9.2%	9.2%	$1,691	$2,002
France	8.9	9.6	1,539	1,978
Germany	8.2	10.5	1,642	2,222
Japan [c]	6.0	7.2	1,082	1,581
United Kingdom	6.0	6.9	957	1,304
United States	12.7	14.2	2,689	3,708

[a] GDP is Gross Domestic Product.
[b] Spending figures have been converted into US dollars.
[c] Japanese data are for 1995.

As you can see in the table below, the United States does not look exceptional in terms of the outcomes of care. After noting that the United States appears to offer its citizens access to care that is comparable to other large industrial countries, Gerald Anderson writes that, in terms of outcomes indicators such as life expectancy and infant mortality, "the United States is frequently in the bottom quartile among the twenty-nine industrialized countries, and its relative ranking has been declining since 1960" (1997). This is not the sort of result that spending far more than the other industrialized countries should give us.

	Life expectancy at birth	
	Males 1995	Females 1995
Canada	75.3	81.3
France	73.9	81.9
Germany	73.0	79.5
Japan[3]	76.4	82.8
United Kingdom	74.3	79.7
United States	72.5	79.2

Source: Anderson, G. F. 1997. "In Search of Value: An International Comparison of Cost, Access, and Outcomes." *Health Affairs* 16 (6): 163–71

1.5 What Does Economics Study?

What does economics study? Economics analyzes the allocation of scarce resources. Although it may appear straightforward, several definitions are needed to understand this sentence. **Resources** include anything that is useful in consumption or production. From the perspective of a manager, resources include the flow of services from supplies or equipment that the organization owns and the flow of services from employees, buildings, or other organizations that the organization hires. A resource is **scarce** if it has alternative uses. These alternative uses might include another use within the organization or use by some other person or organization. Most issues that occupy managers involve scarce resources, so economics has the potential to be useful in nearly all of them.

Economics focuses on rational behavior. That is, it focuses on individuals' efforts to best realize their goals, given their resources. Because time and energy spent in collecting and analyzing the information that is needed to make decisions are scarce resources (i.e., they have other uses), complete rationality is not possible. Everyone uses short cuts and rules to make some choices, and doing so is quite rational, even though better decisions are theoretically possible.

Much of economics is *positive*. That is, economics uses analysis and evidence to answer questions about individuals, organizations, and societies. **Positive economics** *describes* the world, noting, for example, that hospital occupancy rates have fallen in recent years. Positive economics also *explains* the world by proposing hypotheses and assessing how consistent the evidence is with the hypotheses. For example, one might examine whether the evidence supports the conjecture that reductions in direct consumer payments for medical care (measured as a share of spending) have been a major contributing factor in the rapid growth of healthcare spending per person. Although values do not directly enter the realm of positive economics, they do shape it. What questions economists ask (or do not ask) and how they interpret the evidence are surely shaped by values. In this, economists are no different from anyone else.

Other parts of economics are *normative*. **Normative economics** takes two forms. In one, citizens use the tools of economics to answer public policy questions. Usually these questions involve ethical and value judgments (which economics cannot supply) as well as factual judgments (which economics can support or refute). A question such as "Should the Medicare program provide coverage for prescription drugs?" always involves balancing benefits and harms. Economic analysis can help assess the *facts* that underlie the benefits and harms, but it cannot really provide an answer. A second aspect of normative analysis motivates this book. This part tells us how to analyze what we *should do*, given the circumstances that we face. In this part of normative analysis, market transactions give us indications of value that individuals and organizations usually cannot afford to ignore. For example, we may believe that a drug is overpriced, but we must treat that price as a part of the environment and react appropriately if no one will sell it for less. Most managers find themselves in such an environment.

To best realize our goals, given the constraints that we face, economics gives us very explicit guidance that can be broken down into a series of action items.

1. First and foremost, identify the plausible alternatives. Breakthroughs usually occur when someone realizes that there is an alternative to the way things have always been done.
2. Then, explore modifying the standard choice somewhat (e.g., charging a slightly higher price or using a little more of the time of a nurse practitioner).
3. Next, provisionally pick the best choice by finding out the level at which its *marginal benefit* just equals its *marginal cost* (we will explain these terms shortly).
4. Finally, examine whether the total benefits of this activity exceed the total cost. For example, a profit-seeking organization might conclude that a clinic's benefits would be as large as possible if it hired three physicians and two nurse practitioners, but that the clinic's profits would be unacceptably low if it did. Profits would fall still further if the clinic increased or decreased the number of physicians and nurse practitioners, so that is not an option. As a result, the profit-seeking organization would choose to close the clinic.

Let's back up and define some terms to make this discussion clearer. A **cost** is the value of a resource in its next best use. Usually, the next best use of a resource is for someone else to use it instead of us, so the cost is just the price *we* must pay for it. A **benefit** is the value that we place on a desired outcome. We describe this value in terms of our willingness to trade one desired outcome for another. Often, but not always, our willingness to pay money for an outcome is a convenient measure of value. A **marginal** or **incremental** amount is the increased cost that we realize by using more of a resource or the increased benefit that we realize by getting more of an outcome. So, if a 16-ounce soda costs 89 cents and a 24-ounce soda costs 99 cents, the incremental cost of the larger size is (99 - 89)/(24 - 16), or 1.254 per ounce. A rational consumer might conclude that:

- the incremental benefit of the larger soda exceeded its incremental cost and buy the larger size;
- the incremental cost of the larger soda exceeded its incremental benefit and buy the smaller size; or
- the total benefit of both sizes was less than their total cost and buy neither.

(You may recall that complete rationality is not always rational. A consumer with a train to catch might buy an expensive small soda at the station to save time.) It is not an accident that we talked about sodas in defining terms. Buying a soda is both simple and familiar. Healthcare decisions are usually complex and unfamiliar. We suggest, however, that economic analysis will help managers make better decisions about those scarce resources as well.

1.6 Conclusion

Why should healthcare managers study economics? In short, to be better managers. Economics offers a framework that can simplify and improve management decisions. This framework is of value for all managers and is of special value for the many clinicians who must assume leadership roles in healthcare organizations.

References

Anderson, G. F. 1997. "In Search of Value: An International Comparison of Cost, Access, and Outcomes." *Health Affairs* 16 (6): 163–71.

Haugh, R. 1998. "Practice." *Hospitals & Health Networks* 72 (18): 36, 38, 40–41.

AN OVERVIEW OF THE HEALTHCARE SYSTEM

Key Concepts

- Healthcare products are both inputs into health and outputs of the healthcare sector.
- The usefulness of healthcare products varies widely.
- **Marginal analysis** helps managers focus on the right questions.
- Life expectancies have increased sharply in the United States in recent years, but the gains have been smaller and the costs higher than in other industrial countries.
- The outputs of the healthcare sector have changed during the last decade.
- Eight trends continue to reshape the healthcare sector. They are (1) the growth of the healthcare sector; (2) the shrinking share of direct consumer payments; (3) the growth of managed care; (4) the growth of the number of uninsured; (5) the expansion of the outpatient sector; (6) the contraction of the inpatient sector; (7) the growing surplus of hospitals and physicians; and (8) rapid technical change.

2.1 Input and Output Views of Healthcare

This chapter describes the healthcare system of the United States from an economic point of view and defines tools of economic analysis as it introduces the reader to the healthcare system. Our overview looks at the healthcare system from two perspectives. The first, which we call the *input view*, emphasizes the contribution of healthcare to the health of the public. The second, which we call the *output view*, emphasizes the goods and services that the healthcare sector produces. In the language of economics, an **input** is a good or service that is used in the production of another good or service, and an **output** is the good or service that emerges from a production process. It is quite common for a product (both goods and services are considered products) to be both an input and an output. For example, a surgical tool is both an input into a surgery and an output of the surgical tool company. Similarly, the surgery itself can be thought of as the output of the surgical team or as an input into the health of the patient.

2.1.1 The Input View

The input view of the healthcare system stresses the usefulness of healthcare products. From this perspective, healthcare products are neither good nor bad; they are simply tools used to improve and maintain health. The input view is important because it focuses our attention on alternative ways of achieving our goals. For example, products are far from the only inputs into health. Others, such as exercise, diet, or rest, represent alternative ways to improve or maintain health. From this perspective, a switch from medical therapies for high blood pressure to meditation or exercise would be based on the question, "Which is the least expensive way to get the result that I want?"

The input view stresses that the usefulness of any resource, healthcare included, depends on the problem at hand and the other resources available. Whether the health of a particular patient or population will improve as a result of using more healthcare products depends on a number of factors, including the quality and quantity of healthcare products already being used, other health inputs, and the general well-being of the patient or population. For example, the effect of a drug on an otherwise healthy 30-year-old is likely to be quite different from its effect on an 85-year-old who is already taking 11 other medications. Or, increasing access to medical care is not likely the best way to reduce infant mortality in a population that is malnourished and lacks access to safe drinking water, given the more powerful effects of better food and water on health outcomes. Nor is it evident that more medical care is the answer if the question is "What is the best way to use our resources, given that most preventable mortalities are the result of risky behavior?" All of these examples illustrate that the utility of resources varies from situation to situation.

The economic perspective challenges us to examine the effects of *changes* on what we do. This is called **marginal analysis**. A marginal analysis asks questions such as, "How much healthier would this patient or population be if we *increased* use of this resource? How much unhealthier would this patient or population be if we *reduced* use of this resource?" Most management decisions take this form, although they are often more concrete. How much would it cost to increase the chicken pox immunization rate among three-year-olds from 78 to 85 percent, and how much would that reduce the incidence of chicken pox among pre-schoolers? Reasonable answers to these questions will tell us the cost per case of chicken pox avoided, and we can decide if this is how we want to use our resources. These types of questions, although they will be framed differently, are relevant for managers who focus on healthcare products as an output of their organizations. How much will profits rise if we increase the number of skilled nursing beds from 12 to 18? How much would it cost to add a nurse midwife to the practice, and how would this change patient outcomes and revenues? In all of these settings, marginal analysis helps managers focus on the right questions. Figure 2.1 illustrates how variable the effects of medical interventions can be by drawing on the published literature (Tengs 1996) to estimate how many **life years** would be saved by spending $1,000,000 on a particular population. (A life year is one additional year of life for someone, i.e., both one person living for nine additional years and nine persons living for one additional year represent nine life years.) Figure 2.1 tells us that spending $1,000,000 on screening black newborns for sickle cell disease would save more than 4,000 life years; however, spending the same amount on screening non-black, high-risk newborns would save less

Sickle cell screens for black newborns	4,167
Defibrillators in emergency vehicles	2,564
Mandatory motorcycle helmet laws	500
Pneumonia vaccinations for those over age 65	476
Sickle cell screens for non-black, high-risk newborns	9
Sickle cell screens for non-black, low-risk newborns	0

FIGURE 2.1

How Many Life Years Will $1,000,000 Save?

These calculations are based on estimates presented in Tengs, T. O. 1996. "Enormous Variation in the Costeffectiveness of Prevention: Implications for Public Policy." *Current Issues in Public Health* 2 (2): 1317.

than ten life years. Figure 2.1 also reminds us that our attitudes toward health are more complex than we sometimes admit. Spending $1,000,000 on mandatory motorcycle helmet laws would save a few more life years than spending $1,000,000 on vaccinating the over-65 population against pneumonia, yet the helmet law is controversial and the vaccinations are not. Figure 2.1 further reminds us that we do have to make some choices. Screening non-black, low-risk newborns for sickle cell disease saves virtually no life years; however, on a rare occasion, this screening will identify a non-black, low-risk newborn with the disease. We cannot avoid a decision about whether the benefits of this intervention are large enough to justify its very substantial costs. In different ways, these illustrations all remind us that the usefulness of healthcare products varies a great deal.

The input view also stresses that changes in technology or relative prices may change the mix or amount of healthcare products that citizens want to use. For example, lower costs of surgery will increase the number of people who choose vision correction surgery rather than eyeglasses. Conversely, advances in pharmaceutical therapy for coronary artery disease might reduce the rate of bypass graft surgeries (and reduce the attendant hospital stays).

Healthcare managers have not traditionally spent much time on the input view of healthcare. They were charged with running healthcare organizations well, so meditation and other products that their organization did not produce were of little interest. This is changing. Our collective rethinking of the role of health insurance makes the input view very practical. If offering instruction in meditation reduces healthcare use enough, the manager of an insurance plan, a capitated healthcare organization, or the benefits manager of a self-insured employer will find it an attractive option. Increasingly, healthcare managers must be prepared to evaluate a wide range of options.

2.1.2 The Output View

Thinking in new ways does not always mean that the old ways are wrong. The output view of the healthcare sector is more relevant than ever. Producing goods and services efficiently has increased, not decreased, in importance. Struggling with the rising cost of healthcare, those who pay for care are increasingly purchasing it from low-cost producers. At present, third parties (i.e., insurers, governments, and employers) have difficulty distinguishing between care that is inexpensive because it is of inferior quality and care that is inexpensive because it is produced so efficiently; however, their ability to make this distinction is growing. To succeed, managers must lead their organizations to become efficient producers of healthcare products that customers want to do business with. This will be a formidable task in many organizations.

2.2 Health Outcomes

Americans often celebrate their healthcare system as "the best in the world." While parts of the system are indeed superb, it is hard to accept this view overall. In fact, as we indicated in Chapter 1, the American healthcare system has very high costs and relatively mediocre outcomes. Although spending per person is much higher than in any other large, developed country, male life expectancy at birth ranks twenty-second among the 29 members of the Organization for Economic Cooperation and Development, a loose group of industrialized nations. Only Portugal, the Czech Republic, Mexico, Korea, Poland, Hungary, and Turkey trailed the United States (Anderson and Poullier 1999). Given the political decision to subsidize healthcare resources for the elderly, female life expectancy at age 65 might represent a fairer test. On this measure the United States ranked fourteenth. Despite its many areas of excellence, it is difficult to argue that the United States healthcare system is the "best" in the world.

This rather caustic appraisal should not hide the fact that the health of the American public has improved rather dramatically. According to the National Center for Health Statistics (NCHS), between 1960 and 1995, the infant mortality rate fell by 72 percent in the United States, and the death rate among new mothers and mothers-to-be fell even more sharply (1998a). Other death rates have fallen as well. Age-adjusted death rates due to diseases of the heart fell by 53 percent and age-adjusted death rates due to cardiovascular disease fell by 67 percent. Life expectancy at birth rose from 69.7 years in 1960 to 75.8 in 1995, an increase of 6.1 life years per person.

From one perspective, this 6.1 increase in life years represents very impressive performance. From another, it does not compare very well to other industrialized countries. For example, Canadian life expectancy at birth rose from 71.1 in 1960 to 78.3 in 1995, an increase of 7.2 life years per person. Making the comparison look even less favorable, the smaller increase in life expectancy in the United States was realized at about *twice* the cost per life year as the larger Canadian increase. This conclusion rests on a simple marginal analysis in which we compare the change in spending to the change in life expectancy. A concern is that what appears to be higher spending might just be the effects of inflation. To avoid being misled by changes in the value of money, economists use two strategies. The simplest and most reliable strategy reports spending as shares of national income, which economists call Gross Domestic Product. This examination of shares (which we use in Figures 2.4–2.6) removes any effects of inflation. When, as in the current case, we need to compare dollar amounts, we adjust all the spending figures to a common basis. Such inflation-adjusted spending levels are often called **real** spending levels. The price indexes that underlie these adjustments are imperfect, so the adjustments are as well. Consequently, economists are reluctant to make much of small changes in real spending.

To adjust for the effects of inflation, we will multiply spending levels for each year by the value of the Consumer Price Index for the target year (1995 in this case) and divide by the value of the Consumer Price Index for the year in question. The consumer price index equaled 152.4 in 1995 and 29.6 in 1960, so we multiply the 1960 values by 152.4/29.6 to convert them into 1995 terms.

To compare Canadian and U.S. spending we also need to convert them into a common currency. The Organization for Economic Cooperation and Development regularly publishes estimates of spending per person for a number of countries in U.S. dollars, so we can use their data as a starting point (Anderson and Poullier 1999). Converting these figures into inflation-adjusted U.S. dollars, we find that real spending per person in the United States rose from $726 in 1960 to $3,633 in 1995, a 400 percent increase. In contrast, Canadian real spending per person rose from $541 in 1960 to $2,069 in 1995, a 283 percent increase.

Therefore, spending in the United States increased by $2,907 per person per year, while spending in Canada increased by $1,528 per person per year. This very simple marginal analysis does not tell us why costs rose more and life expectancy rose less in the United States, but spending nearly twice as much for a smaller payoff suggests that we are not using our resources wisely.

A Comparison of Health Outcomes in Utah and Nevada

In 1974, Victor R. Fuchs compared health outcomes for residents of Utah and Nevada, noting that, despite their many apparent similarities, residents of the two states were at opposite ends of the health spectrum (Fuchs 1974). Residents of Utah were among the healthiest in the nation; residents of Nevada were among the least healthy. Fuchs argued that the explanation for these health differences "almost surely lies in the different lifestyles of the two states."

Despite major changes in the populations of both states, large differentials persist. Focusing on death rates (the crudest but most accurate measures of health), we see that Nevada's rates remain much higher for adults

One striking change has taken place, however: the two states' infant mortality rates have converged. Fuchs found infant mortality rates in 1974 were more than 35 percent higher in Nevada, much less than the difference in Figure 2.2. Differences in infant mortality rates largely depend on the proportion of children with low birth weights, which is heavily influenced by what individuals do, and survival rates among children with low birth weights, which largely reflects effects of the healthcare system (Guyer et al. 1999). The proportion of children with low birth weights is about 19 percent

FIGURE 2.2

Excess Death Rates in Nevada, 1986–1996

	Male	Female
Under 1 year	3%	−2%
1–19 years	5%	11%
20–44 years	45%	35%
45–64 years	59%	44%
65–84 years	22%	23%
Over 84 years	8%	−1%

Source: Analysis of data from Centers for Disease Control and Prevention. 2000. On-line source [http://wonder.cdc.gov].

higher in Nevada (NCHS 1998a), so the convergence of infant mortality rates appears to reflect improvements in the treatment of infants with low birth weights.

A significant portion of excess mortality in Nevada can be traced to different patterns of alcohol and tobacco use. These lead to much larger age-adjusted death rates for malignant neoplasms of the respiratory system (an uncommon disease among nonsmokers) and for chronic liver disease (including cirrhosis). Only the consequences of alcohol and tobacco abuse are purely medical issues, but how to reduce the consequences of abuse is a classic problem for those taking the input view of healthcare.

These differences in health outcomes are unlikely to be due to differences in healthcare resources. What citizens do (e.g., smoke) and do not do (e.g., exercise) is much more likely to cause these discrepancies, implying that increased use of medical care may not work or may cost much more than alternative interventions. Healthcare is but one tool.

FIGURE 2.3

Excess Age-adjusted Death Rates in Nevada, 1986–1996

	Male	Female
Malignant neoplasms of the respiratory system	136%	239%
Chronic liver disease and cirrhosis	138%	210%

Source: Analysis of data from Centers for Disease Control and Prevention. 2000. On-line source [http://wonder.cdc.gov].

2.3 Outputs of the Healthcare System

In 1997, Americans spent $1.1 trillion on healthcare, meaning that healthcare claimed 13.5 percent of the nation's output (see Figure 2.4). Even though total spending increased by more than $99 billion between 1995 and 1997, healthcare spending actually fell slightly as a share of national income. Even if only an aberration, this small reduction marked the first halt in the rise of healthcare spending as a share of national income since the end of World War II. At this point an alert reader may want to ask, "Why is how much we spend on healthcare interesting? Is there anything wrong with healthcare spending?"

2.3.1 Healthcare Spending

How much we spend on healthcare is interesting for two reasons. First, although an increasing share of national income for healthcare is a world-wide phenomenon, other industrialized countries appear to be realizing larger health gains while spending less than the United States. Second, the rising share of national income spent on healthcare has prompted most governments and employers to question whether the benefits of this increased spending are warranted. If not, there is something wrong with current healthcare spending practices. If the benefits of healthcare spending are smaller than the benefits of using our resources in other ways, a shift would be in order. For example, would we be better off if we had spent somewhat less on educating new physicians and somewhat more on educating new teachers? The **opportunity cost** of a product consists of the goods and services that we cannot have because we have chosen to produce it. The implication is that healthcare need not be bad or worthless for its benefits to be less than its costs, only that it needs to be worth less than some other use of our resources.

Inefficiency represents another concern. It appears that many healthcare outputs could be produced using fewer resources, and some health outcomes could be realized in ways that use fewer resources. If so, healthcare spending represents a problem from the perspective of society. The healthcare system may be wasting resources that have other, more productive uses.

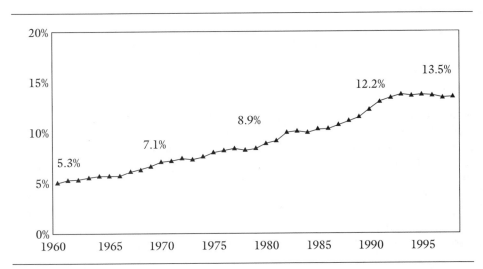

FIGURE 2.4

National Health Expenditures as a Share of GDP

Source: Health Care Financing Administration. 2000. "National Health Expenditures." On-line source [http://www. hcfa.gov/stats]. Accessed 3/9/2000.

2.3.2 The Shifting Pattern of Healthcare Spending

Clearly the mix of outputs of the healthcare sector has changed during the last decade. New technologies and new insurance arrangements are altering what the public buys.

Hospitals produce more than one-third of the output of the healthcare sector; yet this share has fallen during the last decade, even though hospitals' total revenues have increased and they have been expanding into non-traditional markets. For a number of reasons, however, inpatient days have been falling. In addition, other parts of the healthcare sector (most notably the "nondurable medical products" sector and the "other personal healthcare" sector) have been expanding quite rapidly (see Figure 2.5).

To a lesser extent, the services of physicians and dentists have also fallen as a share of total healthcare spending. Again, this is due to the very rapid expansion of other forms of healthcare, not to any decrease in spending for the services of these professionals, which more than doubled between 1987 and 1997.

The largest increases occurred in "other personal healthcare services" and "non-durable medical products." Included in "other personal healthcare services" are home healthcare services; services provided directly to employees by employers; Medicare ambulance services; government spending for healthcare services that do not fall into a standard category; services provided by optometrists, podiatrists, and other licensed practitioners; and services provided by mental health centers, kidney dialysis centers, or substance abuse centers. Home healthcare services rose the fastest of all the sectors, but the other components of "other personal healthcare services" rose almost as fast. Clearly the output of the healthcare sector changed considerably between 1987 and 1997.

"Other non-durable medical products" include prescription drugs, non-prescription drugs, and medical sundries. A **non-durable good** is one that is

FIGURE 2.5
Outputs of the Healthcare Sector

	Amount in millions		Share of the total	
	1997	1987[1]	1997	1987
Hospital care	$371,062	$274,233	34.0%	38.8%
Physician services	217,628	147,132	19.9%	20.8%
Other personal healthcare[2]	138,021	63,574	12.6%	9.0%
Non-durable medical products	108,872	63,299	10.0%	9.0%
Nursing home care	82,774	51,328	7.6%	7.3%
Dental services	50,648	35,806	4.6%	5.1%
Net costs of private health insurance	49,998	26,208	4.6%	3.7%
Public health activity	38,490	19,665	3.5%	2.8%
Research and construction	34,893	25,888	3.2%	3.7%

1. The 1987 figures are in 1997 dollars.
2. Home healthcare, durable medical equipment, and other services.
Source: Health Care Financing Administration. 2000. "National Health Expenditures." On-line source [http://www.hcfa.gov/stats]. Accessed 3/9/2000.

expected to be used up or wear out in a short period of time. Much of the higher output in this category is due to the very rapid growth in prescription drug sales, accounted for by several factors. The first is that as a result of increased insurance coverage for prescription drugs, manufacturers have been able to raise prices. Second, due to rapid innovation, the role of drugs has expanded quite significantly. And third, as care shifts from institutional (i.e., hospitals and nursing homes) to community settings, an increasing proportion of spending on prescription drugs is categorized under non-durable medical products rather than institutional care.

The output of nursing homes has increased somewhat faster than overall healthcare spending, due largely to the growth in the over-85 population. Those over age 85 are the most likely to be residents of nursing homes, even though an increasing number of this aging population continues to live in non-institutional settings. Increased spending has also been fueled by the expansion of skilled nursing care that represents an alternative to lengthy stays in a hospital, and by efforts to upgrade the quality of custodial care. Both of these influences increase the cost per day.

Figure 2.5 also shows "net costs of private health insurance" have increased quite sharply, almost equal to what was spent on dental care in 1997. Health insurance has two components: expenditures on covered services and the net cost of insurance. The net cost of insurance, which includes any profits that the insurance company earns plus the costs of operating the organization, is usually called the *load*. Not surprisingly, given the expanded role of insurance companies in the healthcare system, the net costs of private health insurance have grown faster than overall spending.

Spending on public health activities has also risen significantly, offset by decreases in research and construction.

2.4 Trends Reshaping the Healthcare System

Eight trends continue to reshape the healthcare system of the United States. Most are well known, yet some are so gradual and part of day-to-day operations that even skilled managers tend to ignore them.

1. The growth of the healthcare sector
2. The shrinking share of direct consumer payments
3. The growth of managed care
4. The growth of the uninsured
5. Expansion of the outpatient sector
6. Contraction of the inpatient sector
7. The growing surplus of hospitals and physicians
8. Rapid technical change

2.4.1 The Growth of the Healthcare Sector

The growth of the healthcare sector was a feature of American life for most of the last century, and it has not stopped. Referring back to Figure 2.4, we see that in 1960 healthcare spending claimed only 4.9 percent of national income—in 1997 it claimed 13.5 percent. This continuing expansion has meant two things. One is that a smaller proportion of national income has been available for other purposes. This is a problem only if consumers feel that the benefits of this added spending are smaller than the benefits of spending the money in some other way. The second implication is that a disproportionate share of new jobs has been found in healthcare.

For a typical student, the question of whether this job growth in healthcare will continue to be above average is a more relevant one than musings about the benefits of added healthcare spending. There are two reasons for thinking that the rate of healthcare job creation will slow. First, the expansion of the healthcare sector itself has decreased somewhat in recent years. It is too soon to know if this is a trend, but less expansion would mean slower job growth. Second, changes in the financing system have increased incentives for the healthcare sector to become more efficient. The simplest way to become more efficient is to use hospital care (which is very expensive and very labor-intensive) only when necessary. This trend is already evident and seems likely to continue. Between 1970 and 1995, jobs in the hospital sector grew at about the same pace as jobs in the overall civilian economy (NCHS 1998b).

2.4.2 The Shrinking Share of Direct Consumer Payments

The most consistent force underpinning the evolution of America's healthcare system has been the shrinking share of services that consumers pay for directly. Figure 2.6 shows that consumers paid for 49 percent of healthcare bills in 1960, but only 17 percent by 1997. This sharp decrease, especially between 1960 and 1975, was a result of the introduction of Medicare (in 1966), the conversion of state medical assistance programs into Medicaid (also in 1966), and the expansion of private insurance. **Medicare** is an insurance program run by the Health Care Financing Administration, a federal agency. **Medicaid** is actually the name given to a collection of state programs that meet standards set by the Health Care Financing Administration, but which are run by state agencies. Since 1975, in contrast, the headlines have been quite different. The emphasis in the public sector has been on cost reduction, not expansion. State Medicaid programs shifted beneficiaries into managed care plans, and Medicare adopted new payment systems for hospitals and physicians. Yet despite these efforts to control Medicare costs, its share of total spending rose steadily from 13 percent in 1975 to 19 percent in 1998. Cost controls were more effective for Medicaid, as spending rose very little between 1975 and 1990. Since 1990, however, Medicaid coverage has been significantly expanded, and its share of healthcare expenses rose from 11 percent in 1990 to 15 percent in 1998. Therefore, part of the shift away from direct payment by consumers has been the result of expansion of public programs.

The growth in managed care, the increase in the number of uninsured, and the expansion of payments by consumers have dominated recent discussions of

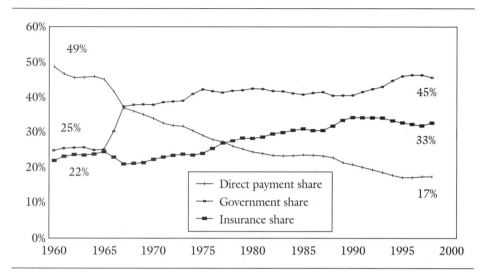

FIGURE 2.6
Consumer,
Insurance, and
Government Shares
of Healthcare
Spending

Source: Health Care Financing Administration. 2000. "National Health Expenditures." On-line source [http://www.hcfa.gov/stats]. Accessed 3/9/2000.

private health insurance. Therefore, a well-informed observer might not understand that the share of healthcare bills paid directly by consumers has continued to drop, because, among those with insurance, coverage has broadened. For example, since 1975, coverage of dental services and pharmaceutical products has become common, and consumers typically pay only part of the bill directly.

2.4.3 The Growth of Managed Care

Insurance has changed considerably in the United States during the last few years. **Managed care** plans have more than doubled their market share among employees. As recently as 1991, less than a third of employees were enrolled in a Preferred Provider Organization (PPO) or a Health Maintenance Organization (HMO). By 1997, however, the trend reversed itself, and more than two-thirds of beneficiaries were enrolled in a PPO or HMO. PPOs largely manage care by securing discounts from hospitals and physicians, while HMOs try to change incentives so physicians have a financial stake in limiting use of services.

This change has been both more dramatic and less dramatic than it seems. It has been more dramatic in that a significant number of fee-for-service (FFS) insurance plans (where providers are paid based on their charges for services) have adopted managed care features like pre-admission certification. Few insurance plans resemble old fashioned, unmanaged indemnity plans any more. It has been less dramatic in that much of managed care does not differ sharply from FFS plans. Virtually all PPO plans and most HMO plans pay providers on a fee-for-service basis. The reason behind this shift to managed care is that many people perceived that the healthcare financing system in place in the United States in 1980 was unworkable. Its costs were too high and its outcomes were too second-rate. New models were needed, and the turmoil of the last decade reflects efforts to develop those models.

2.4.4 *The Growth of the Uninsured*

Increasing numbers of Americans lack health insurance. In 1984, 30 million residents of the United States under age 65 had no health insurance. By 1996 this number had risen to 39 million, representing 16.7 percent of population under age 65 (NCHS 1998c). This number would have risen even faster if Medicaid enrollment had not risen by 11 million.

Increases in the number of the uninsured affect virtually all healthcare organizations. Seriously ill patients without benefits are unlikely to be able to pay their bills. A small number of providers such as free clinics, public health clinics, public hospitals, and university hospitals have traditionally served the bulk of the uninsured. However, there is a real risk that a continuing increase in the number of uninsured patients may, in conjunction with financial pressures from public and private insurers, cause these traditional charity providers to go bankrupt. If so, these patients will not get care, or other providers will face significant demands for charity care.

Most of those without insurance would say that "it costs too much." This response is not very enlightening, because it incorporates at least two very different scenarios. For some, it means that health insurance is worth less than other products. For someone with a low income, good health, few assets, and access to emergency care, insurance is unlikely to be a high priority. In contrast, someone in poor health with a moderate income will be willing to pay substantially more for insurance, but insurance may be very expensive, especially if he or she is not a member of a large group.

Among Americans not eligible for Medicare, nearly two-thirds had insurance through an employer in 1996. There are three main reasons for this. First, the tax laws exclude health insurance premiums from taxable income as long as an employer pays the premiums. This nearly halves the cost of insurance. Second, employment-based insurance sharply reduces insurers' marketing costs. In particular, employment-based insurance allows insurers to spend less to protect themselves against **adverse selection** (where those who anticipate high healthcare bills are much more apt to want coverage than those who anticipate low healthcare bills). Third, Americans have repeatedly rejected health insurance systems run or sponsored by governments. Given the cost advantages of group health insurance, employment-based insurance is the most viable option.

2.4.5 *Expansion of the Outpatient Sector*

In 1980, ambulatory surgeries (those performed on an outpatient basis) represented just over 16 percent of all surgeries. By 1996, ambulatory surgeries represented more than 59 percent of the total. During this same period visits to hospital outpatient departments rose by 92 percent (NCHS 1999). This dramatic shift in the outputs of hospitals overstates the overall expansion of the outpatient sector, but other outpatient services have been expanding as well. Physician contacts per person rose from 5.2 per year in 1985 to 5.8 per year in 1995.

Other outpatient services have expanded even more rapidly. The most dramatic example has been home healthcare services. The number of patients served by home healthcare providers nearly doubled between 1992 and 1996 (NCHS 1998d). Virtually all of this expansion of outpatient care has the effect, intended or not, of continuing the shift out of the inpatient sector.

2.4.6 Contraction of the Inpatient Sector

Contraction of the inpatient hospital sector represents an important trend that is easy to overlook. Figure 2.7 shows that since 1980, days of care per 1,000 persons have fallen by over 50 percent and discharges per 1,000 persons have fallen by more than a third. This contraction, moreover, shows little sign of abating. Areas with high levels of managed care have much lower rates of hospital use than average, and insurers and health systems are just beginning to develop strategies for reducing hospital use still further. In addition, innovations in pharmaceuticals, surgery, and imaging promise to reduce hospital use on a continuing basis.

Many healthcare managers continue to have an inpatient focus. They want to seek improved hospital operations (a worthy aim) to increase the census (an unlikely result). In most areas a better-run hospital will have a census that drops more slowly than less well-run hospitals. Similarly, many managers want to start unprofitable satellite clinics or acquire physician practices (which will be unprofitable after the hospital has assumed management) in the hope of building the inpatient census. In most cases this strategy will fail, as the continuing drop in use of inpatient hospital services will overwhelm any modest increases in referrals that ensue.

2.4.7 The Growing Surplus of Hospitals and Physicians

It appears that the United States has more healthcare capacity than it needs. This is clearest for hospitals. Even though hospital beds per 100,000 residents fell by

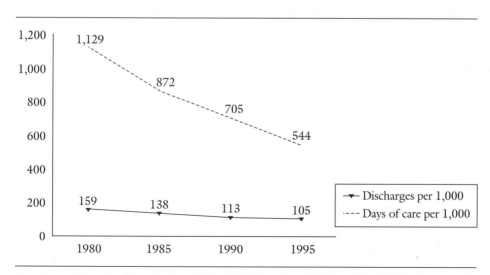

FIGURE 2.7
Hospital Services per 1,000 Persons

Source: National Center for Health Statistics. 1998. *Health, United States, 1998.* Hyattsville, MD: National Center for Health Statistics, Table 88.

23 percent between 1980 and 1995, use of hospitals fell even faster. As a result, hospital occupancy rates have been falling for a number of years. The cost of a vacant bed is a matter of some controversy, but excess capacity clearly costs something.

Although less easy to identify, it is likely that a surplus of physicians is developing. The United States continues to "solve" the healthcare personnel shortage of the 1960s, even though most fields have moved from shortage to surplus. In particular, the number of physicians per 100,000 residents increased by 35 percent between 1980 and 1995. This abundance of physicians, particularly young physicians without established practices, has been one of the factors making the expansion of managed care possible.

2.4.8 Rapid Technical Change

Rapid technical change is pervasive in healthcare. As a result, only luck will rescue management decisions that ignore it. Like every sector of society, healthcare struggles to take advantage of the information revolution. Advances in information processing illustrate the paradox of technical change: lower costs may lead to higher spending. The essence of the information revolution is that the cost of performing a single calculation has dropped precipitously. As a result, many more calculations are possible, and spending on some types of information processing has increased sharply (e.g., computer games) while spending on other types of information processing has plummeted (e.g., inventory management). The challenges of the information revolution are even greater in healthcare than in most sectors. Much of the output of the healthcare sector involves information processing; however, relatively few healthcare workers are highly skilled users of computerized information. Healthcare organizations have lagged behind other service organizations in investing in computer hardware, software, and personnel.

What really sets the healthcare sector apart is the rapid pace of change in other areas: diagnostic and therapeutic outputs are changing even faster than the organizational structure. In some cases (imaging and laboratory services are the most notable examples), technical change is tightly linked to the information processing revolution. In other cases, the links are much looser. For example, advances in information processing speed the development and assessment of new drugs, yet there would be powerful incentives for pharmaceutical innovation even with no change in information processing. Put simply, successful pharmaceutical innovations can be extremely profitable, so investments in pharmaceutical research have been significant.

2.5 Conclusion

At some point during the 1980s, a consensus emerged that the healthcare system of the United States needed to be redirected despite its many triumphs. Underlying this consensus was the recognition that costs were the highest in the world, yet outcomes were not the "best".

How the healthcare system should be redirected is much less clear, and managing under such circumstances is a very stressful occupation. We have suggested, however, that some important trends should guide any organization's objectives. Moreover, there are a number of strategies (like striving to be the low cost producer) that make sense in virtually any environment. In addition to outlining these low risk strategies in the chapters to come, we will also explore strategies for dealing with risk and uncertainty.

References

Anderson, G. F. and J. Poullier. 1999. "Health Spending, Access, and Outcomes: Trends in Industrialized Countries." *Health Affairs* 18 (3): 178–92.

Centers for Disease Control and Prevention. 2000. "Compressed Mortality Database." On-line source [http://wonder.cdc.gov/mortJ.shtml]. Accessed 3/9/2000.

Fuchs, V. R. 1974. *Who Shall Live? Health, Economics, and Social Choice.* New York: Basic Books.

Guyer B., D. L. Hoyert, J. A. Martin, S. J. Ventura, M. F. MacDorman, and D. M. Strobino. 1999. "Annual Summary of Vital Statistics—1998." *Pediatrics* 104 (6): 1229–46.

Health Care Financing Administration. 2000. "National Health Expenditures." On-line source [http://www.hcfa.gov/stats]. Accessed 3/9/2000.

National Center for Health Statistics. 1998a. *Health, United States, 1998.* Hyattsville, MD: National Center for Health Statistics. Tables 23, 45.

National Center for Health Statistics. 1998b. *Health, United States, 1998.* Hyattsville, MD: National Center for Health Statistics. Table 13.

National Center for Health Statistics. 1998c. *Health, United States, 1998.* Hyattsville, MD: National Center for Health Statistics. Table 99.

National Center for Health Statistics. 1998d. *Health, United States, 1998.* Hyattsville, MD: National Center for Health Statistics. Table 133.

National Center for Health Statistics. 1998e. *Health, United States, 1998.* Hyattsville, MD: National Center for Health Statistics. Table 86.

National Center for Health Statistics. 1998f. *Health, United States, 1998.* Hyattsville, MD: National Center for Health Statistics. Table 88.

National Center for Health Statistics. 1999. *Health, United States, 1999.* Hyattsville, MD: National Center for Health Statistics. Table 99.

Tengs, T. O. 1996. "Enormous Variation in the Costeffectiveness of Prevention: Implications for Public Policy." *Current Issues in Public Health* 2 (2): 13–17.

U.S. Department of Labor, Bureau of Labor Statistics. 1999. *Employee Benefits in Medium and Large Private Establishments.* On-line source [http:www.bls.gov/news.release/ebs3.t05.htm]. Accessed 03/13/2000

CHAPTER

3

AN OVERVIEW OF THE HEALTHCARE FINANCING SYSTEM

Key Concepts

- Consumers pay for most medical care indirectly, through taxes and insurance premiums.
- Direct payments for healthcare are often called *out-of-pocket* payments.
- Insurance pools the risks of high healthcare costs.
- Moral hazard and adverse selection complicate risk pooling.
- About 84 percent of the population has medical insurance of some sort.
- Most consumers obtain coverage through an employer-sponsored or government-sponsored plan.
- Insurance as an employment benefit has significant tax benefits.
- Managed care has largely replaced traditional insurance.
- Managed care plans differ quite widely.

3.1 Introduction

3.1.1 Paying for Medical Care

Consumers pay for most medical care indirectly through taxes and insurance premiums. As a result, healthcare managers must understand the structure of private and social insurance programs because these programs will shape much of their organizations' revenues. Managers must also keep sight of the fact that *consumers* ultimately pay for healthcare products, a fact that may be obscured by the complex structure of the U.S. healthcare financing system. A prudent manager will anticipate a reaction when healthcare spending forces higher premiums or taxes, thereby forcing consumers to spend less on other goods and services. Some consumers may drop coverage, some employers may reduce benefits, or some plans may reduce payments. These reactions may not occur if a consensus has emerged in support of increased spending, but managers should still be wary of the profound effects that changes in insurance plans can mean for them. Finally, managers must not limit their thinking to "what insurance will pay for" when considering revenue. Even though the bulk of healthcare firms' revenues represent payments for products covered by insurance plans, consumers do pay directly for some products, especially for those that represent attractive values. In 1997, consumers spent more than $187 billion on healthcare products. Obviously this is a huge market that should not be ignored.

3.1.2 Indirect Spending

Nonetheless, direct consumer spending represents only a fraction of the total spent on healthcare. Figure 3.1 depicts a healthcare market in quite general terms in which consumers pay healthcare providers directly for some services or for part of the costs of others. These direct payments are often called **out-of-pocket** payments. For example, a consumer's payment for the full cost of a pharmaceutical product, for her 20 percent **coinsurance** payment to her dentist, or her eight-dollar **copayment** to her son's pediatrician, are all considered out-of-pocket payments. Insurance beneficiaries make some out-of-pocket payments for services that are not covered by their policy, for services in excess of their policy's coverage limits, or for **deductibles** (requirements that consumers spend a certain amount before their plan pays anything). Another name for out-of-pocket payments is **cost sharing**, a phrase that presumes that indirect payments are the norm. Economics teaches us that a well-designed insurance plan will usually incorporate some cost sharing. We will explore this in detail in our discussion of demand.

The extent of indirect payment distinguishes healthcare markets from most other markets, with three important consequences:

(1) it protects consumers against unexpectedly high healthcare expenses (an intended consequence of most third-party payments);

(2) it encourages consumers to use additional healthcare services (an intended consequence of some third-party payments and an unintended consequence of others); and

(3) it limits the autonomy of consumers in healthcare decision making (an unintended consequence of most third-party payments).

Evidently, the advantages of indirect payment continue to exceed the disadvantages, as indirect payments for healthcare have steadily increased (see Figure 3.2). Both the government and private insurance share of healthcare payments increased substantially during the past century.

FIGURE 3.1

The Flow of Funds in Healthcare Markets

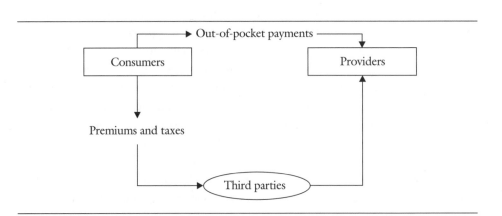

	1929	1960	1997
Inflation-adjusted spending per person	$342	$808	$4,226
Out-of-pocket share	81%	49%	17%
Private insurance share	1%	22%	34%
Government share	14%	25%	45%

FIGURE 3.2

The Growth of Indirect Purchase of Healthcare

Source: U.S. Bureau of the Census. 1975. *Historical Statistics of the United States, Colonial Times to 1970, Bicentennial Edition, Part 2.* Washington, D.C.: U.S. Bureau of the Census.
Health Care Financing Administration. 2000. "National Health Expenditures." On-line source [http://www.hcfa.gov/stats]. Accessed 3/9/2000.

3.1.3 The Uninsured

Most observers regard the rising share of the population without medical insurance as a problem: it rose from 12.9 percent in 1987 to 16.3 percent in 1998, even as out-of-pocket spending continued to fall as a share of total spending. Uninsured consumers enter healthcare markets with two significant disadvantages. First, they must finance their needs from their own resources or those of family, friends, and well-wishers. If these funds are not adequate, they must do without or rely on charity care. The uninsured do not have access to the vast resources of modern insurance companies when large healthcare bills arrive. Second, unlike most insured customers, uninsured customers may be expected to pay list price. The overwhelming majority of insured customers are covered by plans that have secured discounts from providers, indicating that none of the major government insurance plans and few private insurance plans pay list prices for care. While in principle uninsured patients could negotiate discounts for cash payments, this does not appear to be a routine practice.

The uninsured tend to have low incomes. Twenty-three percent of the poor (those with a family income below the federal poverty level) lack health insurance, even though 55 percent are Medicaid beneficiaries. In addition, 27 percent of the near-poor (those with a family income above the poverty level but less than twice the poverty level) are uninsured as well (Kaiser Commission 1998). For many with low incomes, rising healthcare costs have made insurance unaffordable.

The combination of low income and no insurance often creates access problems. For example, 55 percent of uninsured adults reported postponing medical care, compared with 14 percent of privately insured adults, while 24 percent of uninsured adults reported not doing so. Only 4 percent of privately insured adults reported not filling a prescription. Such instances of delaying or foregoing care can lead to even worse health outcomes.

Despite the continuing increase in the number of uninsured consumers, indirect payments continue to represent the largest source of revenue for most healthcare providers. In 1998 they represented 97 percent of payments to hospitals, 84 percent of payments to physicians, and 68 percent of payments to nursing homes (Health Care Financing Administration 2000). Because they are a factor in most healthcare purchases, the structure of indirect payments has a profound influence on the healthcare system and on healthcare organizations.

3.2 What Is Insurance and Why Is It So Prevalent?

3.2.1 What Insurance Does

Fundamentally, insurance pools the risks of healthcare costs, which have a very skewed distribution. Most consumers have quite modest healthcare costs, but a very few incur financially crushing costs. Insurance addresses this problem. Suppose that one person in a hundred had the misfortune to run up $20,000 in medical bills. For simplicity, suppose that no one else had any healthcare bills at all. As long as it is not possible to predict who the unfortunate person will be, a private insurance plan could dramatically reduce the worry associated with this risk. The average bill in our example is $200, as total spending per 100 people will be $20,000. Assuming that everyone is equally apt to confront large healthcare bills, a private firm could offer to pay the healthcare bills of the unfortunate few in exchange for an annual premium of $240 (the $40 extra is our projection of what the firm would charge to cover its selling costs, claims processing costs, and profits). Many consumers would be more than happy to pay $240 to eliminate a one percent chance of a $20,000 bill.

Alas, the world is more complex than this, and such a simple plan would probably not work. To begin with, insurance tends to change the purchasing decisions of beneficiaries. Insured consumers are more likely to use services, and providers no longer feel compelled to limit their diagnosis and treatment recommendations to amounts that individual consumers can afford. These increases in spending that occur as a result of insurance coverage are known as **moral hazard**. Moral hazard can be substantially reduced if consumers face cost sharing requirements, and most contemporary plans have this provision.

3.2.2 Adverse Selection and Moral Hazard

Another, less tractable problem remains. Some consumers, most notably older people with chronic illnesses, are much more likely than average to face large bills. Such consumers would be especially eager to buy insurance. On the other hand, some consumers, most notably younger people with healthy ancestors and no chronic illnesses, are much less likely than average to face large bills. Such consumers would not be especially eager to buy insurance. This is the logic of **adverse selection**: the worst risks are eager to buy insurance, and the best risks are not. At a minimum, the insurance firm would need to carefully assess the risks that individual consumers pose and base their premiums on those risks, a process known as **underwriting**. This would clearly drive up costs. In the worst case, no private firm would be willing to offer insurance to the general public.

In the United States, three mechanisms reduce the effects of adverse selection: employment-sponsored medical insurance, government-sponsored medical insurance, and medical insurance subsidies. In 1998 about 84 percent of the population had medical insurance of some sort. About 25 percent had government-sponsored medical insurance, and just under 60 percent had private medical insurance. (Among Medicare beneficiaries, having both government-sponsored and private Medigap insurance is common. The shares listed here treat those with government-sponsored and private insurance as having government-sponsored insurance). Nine out of ten consumers with private insurance obtained it through their own employer or their spouse's. Few consumers simply bought medical insurance.

3.2.3 Employment and Insurance

Why is the link between employment and medical insurance so strong? To begin with, insurers are able to offer lower prices on employment-based insurance because they have cut their sales costs and their adverse selection risks by selling to groups. It costs only a little more to sell a policy to an entire group of 1,000 than it does to an individual, and relatively few people take specific jobs or stay in them just because of the medical insurance benefits. Medical insurance can also benefit employers. If coverage improves the health of employees or their dependents, workers will be more productive, thereby improving profits for the company. Companies also benefit because workers with employment-based medical insurance are less likely to quit. The costs of hiring and training employees are high, so firms do not want to lose employees unnecessarily. But the most salient factor is likely to be the very substantial tax savings that employment-based medical insurance allows. Medical insurance provided as a benefit by an employer is excluded from Social Security, Medicare, and federal income taxes, and from most state and local income taxes as well. Getting $3,000 in cash instead of a $3,000 medical insurance benefit could easily increase an employee's tax bill by $1,500. It is no wonder, then, that medical insurance is a common fringe benefit and that few consumers who bought their own medical insurance turned down an employment-based plan to do so.

While clearly advantageous from the perspective of individual insurers, employers, and employees, it is less clear that this system is a desirable one from the perspective of society as a whole. The subsidies built into the tax code tend to force tax rates higher, may encourage insurance for "uninsurable" costs like eyeglasses or routine dental checkups, and give employees an unrealistic sense of how much insurance really costs.

The way that most employers frame health insurance benefits further distorts employee choices. In 1997, according to the Center for Studying Health System Change, fewer than 20 percent of private employers allowed employees to choose a plan (1998). Larger employers were much more likely to offer choices, giving about 40 percent of employees a selection. The structure of these choices often encourages employees to choose expensive plans. Most employers pay more when an employee uses a more expensive plan, giving them an incentive to do so. Among employers offering a choice in 1997, 31 percent provided the full cost of the premium as a benefit and 34 percent paid the same share of all plans (which narrows the price difference between high- and low-cost plans). Very few employers share any information about the quality of care offered through different plans or other aspects of plan performance. This makes it unlikely that employees could identify plans with better networks of providers or customer service. For now, at least, it is not likely that consumers have the information that they need to make the health insurance system serve them better.

3.2.4 Medicare as an Example of Complexity

One thing is clear: the health insurance system in the United States is so complex that only a few specialists really understand it. To show why, we will examine the flow of funds built into Medicare. As Figure 3.3 shows, healthcare financing can get quite complicated, even in fairly simple cases. We will start with Medicare beneficiaries. Many pay premiums for Medigap policies that cover deductibles, coinsurance, and other expenses that Medicare does not cover. Like many insurers, Medicare has a deductible. In 1999 the **Part A** deductible was $768 per benefit period and the **Part B** deductible was $100 per year. The most widely applicable coinsurance payments spring from the 20 percent of allowed fees that Medicare beneficiaries must pay for most Part B services. To keep Figure 3.3 simple, we have focused on Medigap policies that reimburse beneficiaries rather than directly paying providers. Beneficiaries with these sorts of policies (and many without Medigap coverage) must make any required out-of-pocket payments directly to providers. Beneficiaries must also pay the Part B premiums that fund 25 percent of this component of Medicare. Like other taxpayers, beneficiaries must also pay income taxes that cover the other 75 percent of Part B costs.

Employers and employees also pay taxes to fund the Medicare system. The most visible of these taxes is the Medicare payroll tax, which is levied on wages to fund Part A (which covers hospital, home health, skilled nursing, and hospice

FIGURE 3.3
The Flow of Funds
in Medicare

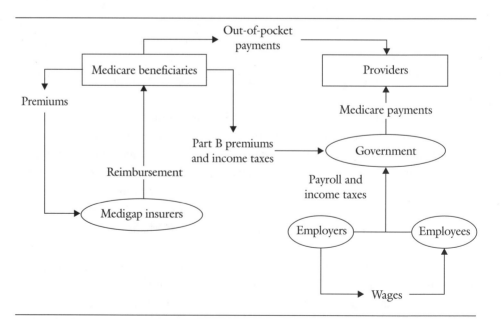

services). In addition, corporation and individual income taxes help fund the 75 percent of Part B costs (outpatient services) that premiums do not cover. The Health Care Financing Administration, the federal agency that operates Medicare, combines these tax and premium funds to pay providers.

Not surprisingly, few taxpayers, beneficiaries, or public officials understand how Medicare is financed. This is not likely to improve policymaking.

Managed Competition at Stanford

In the complex system of healthcare finance of the United States, a major challenge for managers (including those of healthcare organizations) is how to structure benefits so that medical insurance costs are moderate. A key question is whether employees are responsive enough to differences in medical insurance premiums that insurers will have an incentive to offer attractively priced plans. A recent study concludes that employees are quite sensitive to price differences (Royalty and Solomon 1999).

As Figure 3.4 makes clear, employees pay only a part of the total medical insurance premium. This is quite typical. Under the Stanford plan, which is modeled after the managed competition proposals of Stanford economist Alain Enthoven (1984), workers were made responsible for the *entire* difference between the cost of the plan that they chose and Stanford's contribution (which was a percentage of the lowest cost plan). This has tax implications. Employer contributions represent tax-free income for employees, so making employees directly pay a larger share of medical insurance premiums can cost more than might be immediately apparent. On the other hand, plans can be set up to allow employees to make at least some of their direct payments with tax-sheltered dollars. By using tax-sheltered funds, employees in the Stanford plan were able to reduce the after-tax cost of their direct payments for medical insurance by about 29 percent.

More generous coverage costs substantially more (see Figure 3.5). The catastrophic plan, which provides coverage only when healthcare bills become quite large, would cost about $1,550 per year (with the employee directly paying about $30 per year). In contrast, the Point of Service Plan, which offers a broad range of coverage from a loose network of providers would cost about $2,400 per year (with the employee directly paying about $230 per year). Figure 3.5 also shows that more generous plans became relatively more expensive between 1994 and 1995, giving employees an incentive to shift.

As you might expect, employees shifted toward less expensive plans, primarily the more tightly integrated HMOs. Each 10 percent increase in the premium that employees had to pay resulted in a 4 to 7 percent drop in the probability that employees would choose that plan.

FIGURE 3.4

Medical Insurance Premiums in the Stanford Plan

	1994	1995	Percent change
Total monthly premium	$287.20	$274.16	−4.6%
Gross premium paid by employee*	76.10	67.54	−11.9%
Net premium paid by employee*	58.72	50.50	15.1%

*Part of employees' premiums could be paid using pretax dollars, meaning that spending more for medical insurance reduces income taxes. Net premium figures take this into account.
Source: Royalty, A. B. and N. Solomon. 1999. "Health Plan Choice: Price Elasticities in a Managed Competition Setting." *Journal of Human Resources* 34 (1): 1–41.

FIGURE 3.5

Medical Insurance Premiums for Individual Employees

	1994	1995	Percent change
Total monthly premium: point of service plan [1]	$180.00	$172.00	−4.5%
Employee monthly premium: point of service plan	19.12	25.62	29.1%
Total monthly premium: PGP HMO plan[2]	168.00	147.00	−13.3%
Employee monthly premium: PGP HMO plan	18.44	3.40	−137.7%
Total monthly premium: network HMO plan[3]	181.00	165.00	−9.2%
Employee monthly premium: network HMO plan	30.02	19.40	−43.0%
Total monthly premium: catastrophic plan[4]	126.00	120.00	−4.9%
Employee monthly premium: catastrophic plan	2.30	2.24	−2.6%

[1] A Point of Service Plan allows beneficiaries to seek care outside the core network of providers. Doing so increases the required copayment.
[2] A PGP HMO plan requires that beneficiaries get care from physicians in the plan's core group practice. These plans are usually tightly integrated.
[3] A network HMO plan requires that beneficiaries get care from physicians in the plan's network of practices. These plans are usually loosely integrated.
[4] A catastrophic plan provides no benefits until beneficiaries spend a large amount of money.
Source: Royalty, A. B. and N. Solomon. 1999. "Health Plan Choice: Price Elasticities in a Managed Competition Setting." *Journal of Human Resources* 34 (1): 1–41.

3.3 The Rise of Managed Care

Traditional open-ended fee-for-service plans (of which pre-1984 Medicare was a classic example) have three basic problems. First, they encourage providers and consumers to use covered services as long as the *direct* cost to consumers is less than the direct benefit. Since the total cost of care is much greater, consumers may well use services that are worth much less than they cost. In addition, open-ended fee-for-service plans discourage consumers from using uncovered services, even highly effective ones. Finally, much of the system of consumer and provider incentives is accidental, in that the prices paid by consumers and the prices received by providers do not reflect provider costs or consumer valuations.

Given the origins of traditional medical insurance, these incentives make good sense. Medical insurance was started by providers, largely in response to the inability of consumers to afford expensive services and the unwillingness of some consumers to pay their bills once services had been rendered. The goal was to cover the costs of services, not to provide care in the most efficient manner possible or to improve the health of the covered population.

What is managed care? It is a collection of insurance plans with only one real common denominator: a perception that traditional, open-ended, fee-for-service insurance plans are no longer tenable. A traditional open-ended plan covered all services if the service was covered by the contract and if a provider, typically a physician, was willing to certify that it was "medically necessary." Payment to the provider was based on the charges submitted. Hospital care was "free" from the perspective of physicians, and usually did not cost the patients very much. Generous coverage of hospital services and limited coverage of some outpatient services meant that extensive use of costly hospital services served the needs of both patients and physicians quite well, while driving healthcare costs higher and higher.

At present, managed care comes in four basic forms: PPOs, staff and group model HMOs, IPA HMOs, and POS HMOs. We will briefly describe each of these forms of managed care organizations. Be forewarned, however: there is almost always an exception to every generalization that we make in the next paragraph, and will have only scratched the surface of the heterogeneity of managed care plans.

The most common form of managed care organization is a Preferred Provider Organization (PPO). All PPOs negotiate discounts with a panel of hospitals, physicians, and other providers. After that, PPOs diverge. Some have small panels, while some employ other techniques, such as requiring that care be approved by a primary care gatekeeper. The variability of PPOs makes their common label rather suspect, but they are far less diverse as a group than Health Maintenance Organizations (HMOs). Traditional HMOs are structured around large group practices. Group model HMOs contract with a small number of groups, whereas staff model HMOs directly employ physicians. Group model HMOs usually capitate physician groups (i.e., pay physicians per beneficiary enrolled with them), where staff model HMOs usually pay salaries. These HMOs still exist, but they are expensive to set up and make sense only for large numbers of enrollees. Much of the expansion of HMOs has been fueled by the growth of Independent Practice Association HMOs, or IPAs. These plans contract with both large and small groups of physicians, and even with solo practice physicians. These contracts can assume many forms. Physicians can be paid per service (as PPOs usually do) or per enrollee (as group model HMOs usually do). IPAs also pay hospitals and other providers using a wide variety of techniques. The other form of HMO is called a Point of Service (POS) HMO. These plans resemble a combination of a PPO and an IPA. Unlike an IPA, they cover non-emergency services provided by non-network providers, although copays are higher. Unlike a PPO, they pay some providers using methods other than discounted fee-for-service.

Clearly, we are living through the messy process of the evolution of managed care. Exactly where this process will lead is not clear. Wiser observers have been repeatedly wrong (or at least right too soon). The implication for managers is that change represents the only guaranteed component in the healthcare financing system. Whatever it is, managed care has exploded on the healthcare scene. As we noted in Chapter 2, managed care has become the most common form of insurance in the United States today.

Managed care plans seek to change the incentives created by these open-ended fee-for-service plans in several ways by:

- Changing financial incentives for providers, as do Medicare's DRG system and the global payment systems of some HMOs.
- Changing financial incentives for consumers, including lower copays for preventive services and higher copays for branded pharmaceuticals.
- Using their market power to secure advantageous contracts, such as plans negotiating provider discounts.
- Creating bureaucratic structures that reduce use of low-valued care and increase use of high-valued care (known as **utilization review plans**).
- Selecting providers with below-average costs and above-average outcomes. These sorts of arrangements are most common in tightly integrated plans that contract with a limited number of hospitals and physician groups. In turn, the physician groups deal with a limited number of insurance plans. In the most tightly integrated plans, physicians only treat patients covered by one plan. More typically, physicians treat patients insured by hundreds of plans.

How Insurance Plans Manage Care

What do managed care plans do to alter patterns of care that traditional insurance plans do not? Rather less than you might imagine, according to a recent study that focused on managed care from the perspective of physicians (Remler 1997). While the study emphasized HMOs, which manage care more strictly than PPOs or POS plans, physicians were asked about the percentage of all patients who were affected by a managed care technique, whether the patient was in a managed care plan or not.

Utilization review was common, but only weakly linked to the market share of HMOs. For example, reviews of hospital length of stay were common. Among physicians in areas with high HMO penetration, insurers reviewed it for 57 percent of patients. In areas with low HMO penetration, length of stay was reviewed for 60 percent of patients. Similarly, insurers reviewed the appropriateness of treatment for 42 percent of patients in high HMO penetration areas and for 40 percent of patients in the low areas.

Although much in the news, denials of coverage were uncommon and usually reversed on appeal. For example, the initial denial rate for hospitalization was 3.4 percent, but two-thirds of these denials were reversed. The pattern was much the same for surgical procedures. The initial denial rate for hospitalization was 3.7 percent, with two-thirds reversed. Referrals to particular specialists were more commonly denied. The initial denial rate was 5.7 percent, and just more than two-fifths of these denials were supported. Denials of behavioral health referrals were more common than other types, but were not the norm. Three percent of referrals for mental health services were sustained, as well as 2.8 percent of substance abuse referrals to specific providers. In fact, as Figure 3.6 shows, a broad range of managed care techniques appear to be less common and less closely linked to HMO penetration than one might anticipate.

FIGURE 3.6

Shares of Patients Affected by Managed Care Techniques

	HMO penetration	
	High	Low
Protocols and guidelines	19%	12%
Discounted fees	43%	40%
Provider profiling	19%	11%
Member of a restricted panel	33%	21%
Gatekeeper	22%	12%

Source: Remlar et al. 1997. "What Do Managed Care Plans Do to Affect Care? Results from a Survey of Physicians." *Inquiry* 34 (3): 196–204.

3.4 Payment Systems

Until quite recently, virtually all healthcare providers were paid on a simple fee-for-service basis. Managed care plans have begun to experiment with alternative payment arrangements, which is important in that different payment systems create different incentive systems for providers. It is clear that differences in financial incentives lead to different patterns of care, so the power of changing incentives should not be underestimated (Hellinger 1996). In contracting with insurers or providers, managers need to recognize the strengths and weaknesses of different systems.

3.4.1 The Four Basic Payment Methods

There are only four basic payment methods: *salary, fee-for-service, case-based,* and *capitation.* Each can be modified by the addition of incentive payments, so the number of possible payment methods can become quite large.

Salary and fee-for-service payments are common. A **salary** is a payment per period of time. As such, it is not directly linked to output. Salaries are most common when productivity is difficult to measure (as it is for an academic physician) or when the incentives created by fee-for-service payments are seen as undesirable (as they are in some HMOs). Historically, however, most physicians in the United States have been paid on a **fee-for-service** basis. In this system, each physician has a schedule of fees and expects to be paid that amount for each unit of service provided.

Case-based and capitation payments may not be familiar, so we will briefly describe them. As you might expect, a **case-based** payment makes a single payment for all of the covered services associated with an episode of care. Medicare's DRG system is a case-based system for hospital care, although it does not include physicians' services or post-hospital care. In essence, case-based payments are fee-for-service payments with the "service" defined very broadly. **Capitation** represents a payment per beneficiary enrolled with a physician or organization. Capitation can be thought of as a salary that varies with the number of customers.

3.4.2 Advantages and Disadvantages

Each of the four basic payment methods has advantages and disadvantages. *Salaries* are quite simple and incorporate no incentives to overuse care. By themselves, however, salaries create only weak incentives for high levels of effort or exemplary service. In addition, salaries give providers incentives to use resources other than their time and effort to meet their customers' needs. In the absence of incentives not to, salaried providers may well seek to refer substantial numbers of patients to specialists, urgent care clinics, or other sources of care. *Capitation*, as we have noted, incorporates many of the same incentives as a salary, but with two important differences. One is that capitation payments drop if customers defect, which creates a stronger, more immediate incentive than salary to please customers. The other is that capitation arrangements often put providers or organizations at risk for costs other than their own time and effort. Since profits rise if these other costs fall, capitation encourages greater efficiency, referral to other providers, or undertreatment.

In contrast, *fee-for-service* payments create powerful incentives for high levels of effort and service. In fact, it may well result in over-treatment of insured consumers, by making it profitable to recommend services whose costs exceed their benefits, as long as the benefits exceed the consumer's out-of-pocket cost. These incentives can complicate efforts to control costs, as attempts to impose or negotiate lower rates are likely to be met with efforts to "unbundle" care by billing separately for procedures or tests that may once have been part of the basic service. *Case-based* rates combine many of the features of fee-for-service and capitation. The strong incentives to provide service remain, as do those to increase profits by reducing costs that are included in the case rate. Costs can be reduced by improving efficiency, shifting responsibility for therapy to "free" sources, and narrowing the definition of a case. The challenge is to keep providers focused on improving efficiency, not on "gaming" the system.

Any of these four basic methods can be significantly modified by bonuses and penalties. A base salary for a hospitalist plus a bonus for reducing inpatient days in selected cases does not much resemble a straight salary contract. Similarly, a capitation plan with bonuses or penalties for customer service standards (e.g., a bonus for returning more than 75 percent of after-hours calls within 15 minutes) has incentives quite different from plain capitation.

3.4.3 *Capitation Loses Ground*

A few years ago, everyone believed that capitation would become the dominant method of payment. Experience suggests, however, that few providers (or insurers, for that matter) have the administrative skills or data that capitation demands. In addition, the financial risks can be quite substantial. Few providers have enough capitated patients for variations in average costs to cease being worrisome, and capitation payments are seldom risk adjusted (i.e., increased when spending can be expected to be higher than average). These considerations have dampened the enthusiasm of most providers for capitation, and insurers have come to realize that it is not the "cure all" method they once believed it to be. Coupled with the recognition that providers have many ways other than becoming more efficient to reduce their costs, insurers have lost interest as well. Thus far, fee-for-service payments to providers remain the norm, even in most HMOs. What compensation arrangements will look like in ten years is yet to be seen.

3.5 Conclusion

The last two decades have seen the virtual disappearance of traditional, open-ended insurance plans. Even those that are not called managed care plans usually have incorporated some managed care components in an effort to keep premiums down. Yet the explosion of managed care plans should not hide the fact that most consumers are in plans that are not very "managed." Most consumers are enrolled in PPO or POS plans that pay providers in familiar ways, and most providers are not really part of an organized delivery system.

Yet the healthcare financing system of the United States appears to be changing dramatically. The share of spending paid for directly by consumers has continued to drop, even as the proportion of consumers without health insurance continues to rise. Among those with insurance, coverage has gotten more complete and the share of spending financed by taxes has continued to rise. Cost sharing by patients has become a routine part of health insurance plans even as other forms of direct spending have decreased.

No one really knows where the healthcare system of the United States is headed. The process of change substantially increases the risks that healthcare managers must face. The next chapter will introduce the basics of how to manage risks. Of course, becoming the most efficient producer is a strategy that works in virtually all environments, and we will develop tools for doing that in the chapters to follow.

References

Center for Studying Health System Change. 1998. "How Widespread is Managed Competition?" *Data Bulletin* 12: 1–3. [http://www.hschange.com/databull].

Enthoven, A. 1984. "A New Proposal to Reform the Tax Treatment of Health Insurance." *Health Affairs* 3 (1): 21–39.

Health Care Financing Administration. 2000. "National Health Expenditures." On-line source [http://www.hcfa.gov/stats]. Accessed 3/9/2000.

Hellinger, F. J. 1996. "The Impact of Financial Incentives on Physician Behavior in Managed Care Plans: A Review of the Evidence." *Medical Care Research and Review* 53 (3): 294–314.

Kaiser Commission on Medicaid and the Uninsured. 1998. *Uninsured in America, Chart Book*. On-line overview. [http://www.kff.org].

Remler, D. K., K. Donelan, R. J. Blendon, G. D. Lundberg, L. L. Leape, D. R. Calkins, K. Binns, and J. P. Newhouse. 1997. "What Do Managed Care Plans Do to Affect Care? Results from a Survey of Physicians." *Inquiry* 34 (3): 196–204.

Royalty, A. B. and N. Solomon. 1999. "Health Plan Choice: Price Elasticities in a Managed Competition Setting." *Journal of Human Resources* 34 (1): 1–41.

U.S. Bureau of the Census. 1975. *Historical Statistics of the United States, Colonial Times to 1970, Bicentennial Edition, Part 2*. Washington, D.C.: U.S. Bureau of the Census.

U.S. Bureau of the Census. 2000. *Health Insurance Coverage: 1998*. On-line source. [http://www.census.gov/hhes/hlthins/hlthin98/hi98tl.html.] Accessed 3/15/2000.

DESCRIBING, EVALUATING, AND MANAGING RISK

Key Concepts

- Clinical and managerial decisions typically entail uncertainty about what will happen.
- Often decision makers have imprecise estimates of the probabilities of various outcomes.
- Decision making in the face of risk involves describing risky outcomes, evaluating risky outcomes, and managing risk.
- Managing risk involves insuring or diversifying.

4.1 Introduction

Clinical and managerial decisions typically entail risk. Most of the time important information is missing when the time to make a decision arrives. At best, one knows what the outcomes can be and what the probability of each outcome is; at worst, one lacks virtually any information about outcomes and probabilities. The challenge for managers is to identify the risks that are worth analyzing, the risks that are worth taking, and the best strategy for dealing with those risks.

Decision making when outcomes are uncertain has three components: describing risky outcomes, evaluating risky outcomes, and managing risk. Because uncertainty is central in many areas, decision making is similar when dealing with real investments (e.g., buildings, equipment, or training), financial investments (e.g., stocks, bonds, or insurance), and clinical decisions (e.g., testing and therapy). In all of these instances we recommend the same techniques for describing, evaluating, and managing risky outcomes. Other techniques, such as hedging one's bets and aggressively monitoring uncertain situations, are also valid; therefore, our discussion will apply to a wide range of choices.

Risk and Capitation

With varying amounts of enthusiasm, healthcare providers are assuming risk by accepting **capitation** (a fixed payment per beneficiary regardless of the amount of service provided). Because of this, Alison Cherney points out, providers must begin to think systematically about risk and uncertainty (1996). She explains that risk depends on the probability of a loss and on the size of that loss. For example, the probability of a beneficiary requiring a liver transplant may be only one in 10,000. Yet this remains a major risk, because the cost of a liver transplant is so large.

In evaluating a capitation contract, providers face three separate problems. First, there may be considerable uncertainty about utilization rates of some services. Health plan data may inadequately describe the risks that providers face, especially for out of network services. Second, the demographics of the plan's population may change from year to year, shifting utilization patterns and affecting the profitability of last year's capitation rates. Third, except for very large groups of patients, the actual incidence of illness may differ from the underlying statistical rates (i.e., two patients may need liver transplants in the same year, even though the rate is actually only one in 10,000).

Cherney notes that a variety of methods can help providers reduce risk. They can purchase stop-loss insurance, which covers very large claims. Unfortunately, stop-loss insurance is seldom available for new plans, but providers can often negotiate clauses that exclude certain high-cost cases or include provisions for outlier cases. Another common strategy for limiting risk is a risk band, which adjusts the capitation rate when utilization is higher or lower than expected. Risk bands are often first steps in the process of moving toward a fixed capitation rate. Providers can also control risk by **carving out** some services. This means that another provider is responsible for the care of some patients and that the capitation payment no longer covers them. For example, a local mental health center might care for patients with serious mental illnesses or a rehabilitation facility might care for patients who have had strokes.

All methods to reduce risk will also reduce expected profit; however, the final rate negotiated should have profit potential. If not, both parties have made a mistake. It is in neither side's interest for the provider to lose money on the contract. The insurer's real hope is that the provider will manage care so well that the provider, the insurer, and the beneficiaries all win.

4.2 Describing Risky Outcomes

The first step in making any decision is to describe the probabilities and values of the possible outcomes and to calculate any descriptive statistics that are helpful. Only the calculations are easy.

Description begins with an assessment of the probabilities of the possible outcomes. Ideally, these probabilities would be soundly based on evidence about the frequencies of different outcomes. For example, if 250 of 1,000 patients reported nausea after taking a medication, a good estimate of the probability of nausea would be 0.25 (250/1,000). The idea of a probability seems clearest in these circumstances, when an **objective probability** based on frequencies makes sense. More often, however, decisions are based on **subjective probabilities**, the decision maker's perception of how likely an outcome is. In some cases decision makers simply have incomplete data or the data may not fit. For example, even if a careful study of a drug in a population of men over the age of 18 finds that the probability of nausea is 0.25, what value should we use for a sample of women over the age of 65? In other cases, individuals may feel that population frequencies do not apply to them (i.e., someone who believes he has a "cast iron stomach" may think that his probability of nausea is much less than 0.25).

In practice, decision makers routinely use subjective probabilities, believing their personal assessments of the chances that various outcomes will be realized. Unfortunately, these subjective probabilities are often wrong, even when made by highly trained clinicians or experienced managers. Studies have found physicians' overestimatations of the probability of skull fractures, cancer, pneumonia, and streptococcal infections. And managers are notorious for being overly enthusiastic in their forecasts of how well new projects will be executed and received. For a variety of reasons, humans appear to be rather bad probability calculators. Therefore, simply providing data about population frequencies can significantly improve choices. For example, even if you believe that your hospital is less likely than average to lose money on the primary care practices it has just purchased, knowing that the overwhelming majority of hospitals *has* lost money tells you that you are still apt to suffer losses as well.

In many cases, moreover, an honest assessment of the probabilities results in broad generalizations, not a point estimate of probabilities. A manager may only be able to say, "I think this scenario is more likely than that one." This is still useful information, as general impressions about how likely a scenario is can powerfully clarify what should be done.

4.3 Valuing Outcomes

The next step is to describe and value possible outcomes. In this chapter we will focus on outcomes that have money values, typically profits. This is usually quite challenging. Skilled analysts will routinely get different answers when asked to calculate how much a therapy will cost under well-defined circumstances. When asked to forecast costs and revenues for a new project, with all its attendant uncertainties, the range of plausible forecasts increases dramatically. While it may be possible to improve forecasts somewhat, they will never be more than educated guesses. This must be reflected in your decision-making process.

As you can imagine, the problems mount when no simple measurement system, like profits, exists. How valuable is a new surgical procedure that reduces the chance of abdominal scarring from 0.12 to 0.08, but reduces the chance that the operation will succeed from 0.68 to 0.66? Any time that outcomes differ in a number of ways, valuation becomes a challenge. Even though scholars have made considerable progress in evaluating complex outcomes, considerable uncertainty remains. We will tackle this valuation problem in more detail in Chapter 12.

4.3.1 Calculating Descriptive Statistics

Calculating descriptive statistics is the final step in the process of describing outcomes. The most common statistic is the **expected value** or average. To calculate an expected value, first multiply the value of each outcome and its probability of occurrence, then add the resulting products.

Suppose, for example, your organization is contemplating buying a skilled nursing facility for $1,000,000. At present, the facility is barely breaking even. One of your young managers, however, has identified a number of operational improvements and product line changes that she forecasts will boost profits to $125,000, representing a 12.5 percent return on equity (125,000/1,000,000). While accepting the reasonableness of the manager's proposals, a consultant has pointed out that there is at least one chance in three that there will be a further reduction in government rates. If this happens, the facility could earn no more than $50,000. The consultant also states that, in his experience, ambitious proposals to increase profits fall short about half the time. He estimates that to be realistic, you should anticipate earning about two-thirds of the forecast return on equity in these situations.

This level of precision (e.g., "about half the time") is representative of the reliability of managerial forecasts. The forecast is tenuous at best, yet managers must make a choice. In many cases, calculating the expected return on equity and then doing a sensitivity analysis will help them.

Formally, an expected value equals $P_1X_1, + P_2X_2, + \ldots + P_nX_n$, with P_i representing the probability that an outcome will occur and X_i representing the value of that outcome. An expected value differs from a garden variety average because not all the probabilities equal $1/n$. In this case the expected return on equity is 7.8 percent. This is just equal to $12.5\% \times 0.335 + 5.0\% \times 0.335 + 8.3\% \times 0.165 + 3.3\% \times 0.165$.

4.3.2 Visual Representations of Information

Good decisions usually require more information than just an expected value, since the expected value is typically not an outcome that will actually occur. Most decision makers find that making a list of the best and worst outcomes, as well as the most likely one, is valuable. Decision makers often find a well-designed graph is of more value than a calculation in helping them to understand their choices. Finally, remember that your estimates are just that: writing down an estimate does not make it more reliable. The less mathematically sophisticated your target audience, the more you need to emphasize that forecasts are necessarily imprecise.

A very simple way to represent information about a choice is to create a decision tree, which visually links a decision maker's choices with the outcomes that are likely to result. It is called a tree because the possible outcomes branch out from a choice. For the analyst, much of the value lies in the process of constructing the decision tree, as it highlights his or her perception of what will happen and where the information is weakest. In addition, many people find that examining a decision tree helps then understand the issues involved, as it lays out the best estimates of the cost or payoff and the probability associated with each possible outcome. As you can see clearly in Figure 4.1, the worst-case forecast is for a return on equity of 3.3 percent, which is less than ideal, but not a catastrophe. Similarly, the best-case forecast is for a return on equity of 12.5 percent, which is good, but not superb. As is usually the case, laying out the decision tree helps clarify the situation by making the probability and return on equity estimates explicit. It does not tell managers what decision to make, especially when the alternatives are not yet clear.

Calculating the expected values of alternatives is sometimes called "rolling back" a decision tree, which represents no more than calculating its expected value. In Figure 4.1, the expected return on equity (ROE) is 7.8 percent.

4.3.3 Estimating the Variability of Outcomes

Estimates of the variability of outcomes can be useful for making comparisons. Variability is typically measured by listing the range of possible values or the standard deviation (or variance if you prefer your numbers larger). If you are not comparing outcomes, the standard deviation is not helpful. In contrast, the range can convey useful information even if you are not comparing outcomes, as

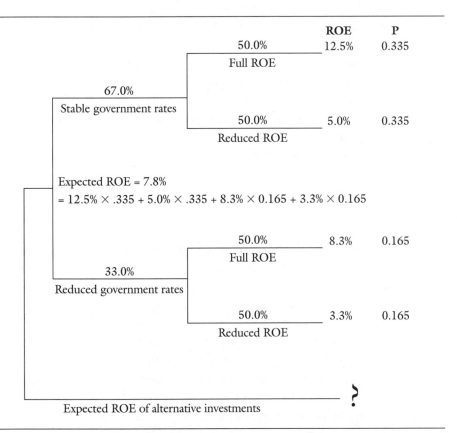

FIGURE 4.1

A Decision Tree for the Nursing Facility Purchase Decision

it lets you see the best-case and worst-case scenarios. To know whether a risk is worth taking, you need to know the size of both the risk and the potential payoff. Few people will want to take much risk if the best possible payoff is small or if the worst payoff is disastrous. On the other hand, if the best payoff is large, some people will be willing to accept significant risks.

To calculate a standard deviation, first multiply the squared difference between value of each outcome and the expected value and its probability of occurrence, then add the resulting products and find the square root of the sum. In our example, the standard deviation is $(12.5\% - 7.8\%)^2 \times 0.335 + (5.0\% - 7.8\%)^2 \times 0.335 + (8.3\% - 7.8\%)^2 \times 0.165 + (3.3\% - 7.8\%)^2 \times 0.165)^{0.5}$ or 3.7 percent. The variance is just the square of the standard deviation. (These calculations are easy to do on a spreadsheet. Simply entering the formula $+ X^2$ in QuattroPro or Lotus $(= X^2$ in Excel) calculates a square. The formulas $+ X^{0.5} (= X^{0.5}$ in Excel) calculate a square root. Many calculators also can do these computations.)

A standard deviation or variance has meaning only when comparing actions. If two outcomes have similar expected values, the one with the higher standard deviation carries a higher risk, as a larger standard deviation means that the bad outcomes are either more likely or much worse. For example, a risky project that has a 50 percent chance of a return of 19.6 percent and a 50 percent chance of a return of −4 percent also has an expected return of 7.8 percent. The standard deviation for this project is not 3.7 percent, but 11.8 percent, confirming its higher risk.

Remember, however, that the point of these calculations is to improve analysis. That analysis must include an understanding of the size of the risk, how likely it is, and whether it is worth taking. If your target audience, which might include members of the board or non-financial managers, gets buffaloed by your analysis and does not really understand these issues, the analysis has failed. You have not gotten useful feedback from your audience, and the risk is entirely yours. While managers *may* get fired for taking risks that are understood and approved, they generally *do* get fired for those that are not.

4.4 Risk Preferences

Risk preferences may influence choices. A **risk seeking** person prefers more variability. Someone who gambles in a casino is usually a risk seeker, because the expected payoff from a dollar bet will always be less than a dollar because of taxes and the casino's take. Likewise, a patient with an expected life span of 18 months with standard therapy may be a risk seeker because he prefers a therapy that reduces his life expectancy to only 13 months, but increases his chances of a significant recovery. The manager of a nearly bankrupt business is also likely to be a risk seeker, since taking chances, even ones with low expected payoffs, may be the only way to survive.

A **risk neutral** person does not care about variability and will always choose the outcome with the highest expected value. Large organizations with substantial reserves can afford to be risk neutral. For example, a firm with $400 million in cash reserves will probably not buy fire insurance for a $200,000 clinic. If the expected loss is $4,000 per year (reflecting a 2 percent chance of a total loss), the organization's fire insurance will cost at least $4,400 because of processing costs and insurer profits. On average, the firm will have higher profits if it does not insure this risk, especially since it can afford not to do so. Spending $200,000 for a new clinic will not significantly decrease the organization's reserves.

A **risk averse** person avoids variability and will sometimes choose strategies with smaller expected values to avoid risk. An individual who buys health insurance is likely to be risk averse, because the expected value of her covered expenses will usually be less than the premium. Insurance premiums must cover the insurer's expected payout, its cost of operation, and some return on invested capital. Unless the expected benefits (the insurer's expected payouts) have been incorrectly estimated, the insurer's costs and profits will push insurance premiums above expected losses. By definition, someone who will pay this is risk averse.

4.5 Decision Analysis

Formal decision analysis has three steps, only one of which is difficult. The steps are setting up a decision tree, identifying the alternative with the largest expected value, and using sensitivity analysis to assess the analysis. Creating a decision tree is by far the hardest and most important part of decision analysis. It is here that most insights can be gained and that most mistakes are made. To set up a decision tree, one needs to

1. Carefully define the problem. This is often more difficult than it sounds.
2. Identify the alternative courses of action. Serious mistakes are often made here.
3. Identify the outcomes associated with each alternative.
4. Identify the sequence of events leading to final outcomes. This sequence may include choices and chance events.
5. Calculate the probability of each outcome.
6. Calculate the value of each outcome.

Be advised that each of these steps can be more difficult than it sounds. Therefore, the first decision is often whether to even do a decision analysis or not. Only occasionally will it be prudent to carefully analyze a decision, but avoiding one or two major mistakes can make decision analysis worthwhile.

4.6 Sensitivity Analysis

Any time it is worthwhile to set up and solve a decision tree, it is worthwhile to do a sensitivity analysis. A sensitivity analysis simply substitutes different, but plausible, values for the values in a decision tree. It is always helpful to know how sensitive the results are to minor changes in the data. The data are never perfect, and it would not make sense to act as though they were.

The decision tree for the nursing facility purchase tells us that the key issue is whether its manager can actually realize the operational improvements and product line changes that she contemplates. If she can, the return on equity will be no less than 8.3 percent, no matter what Medicare does. A sensitivity analysis tells us that if she can realize about 70 percent of her projected gains, she will have an expected return on equity of 7 percent. This gives rise to the question, "What could we do to increase the odds of the full improvement?" The sensitivity analysis has told us that we can fall somewhat short of the manager's prediction and still hit our target rate of return.

4.7 Managing Risk

There are really only two strategies for managing risk: risk sharing and diversification. Buying an insurance policy is the obvious way to do share risk, although many joint ventures can serve essentially the same function. Insurance consists of paying a fee to induce some other organization to share risks; joint ventures share costs and profits with partners. Diversification can take a number of forms. Horizontal integration (creating an organization that can offer the full spectrum of health care services) is one diversification strategy, as it is likely that at least some aspects of healthcare will be profitable, no matter what the environment. Joint ventures and options are other, less-known ways of managing risk. All of these strategies limit potential losses and, of course, potential profitability.

Joint Ventures Help Manage Risk

Joint ventures and options are common in the biotechnology and pharmaceutical fields. For example, in early 1999, Inspire Pharmaceuticals of Durham, North Carolina announced a partnership with Santen Pharmaceutical of Osaka, Japan. Inspire gets cash and potential royalty earnings. Santen gets access to new technology, and exclusive rights to market in Japan and other Asian countries, a drug called INS365, which is designed to treat dry eyes. In effect, Santen has, for $6.25 million, bought an option to develop and market INS365. (It does not have to develop and market INS365. It merely has the opportunity to do so.) For Santen, this is a small risk with a large profit potential. Inspire, a tiny startup, has sold this option to help fund its research. For Inspire, this is a large risk that it would like to share with others. Furthermore, should the product be successful, Inspire would need a distribution partner in Japan.

In a similar venture that was announced several days earlier, a German pharmaceutical firm paid Medarex, of Annadale, New Jersey, $1.5 million for the option to negotiate for worldwide licensing rights (Medarex would retain U.S. rights). In both of these cases, small firms are sharply reducing their risks by selling to other companies the rights to sell products outside the United States. Both of these joint ventures reduce one party's risk and potential gains while increasing the risk and potential gains of the other party. In each case, the party that accepts more risk is better able to do so, either because of specialized expertise or because of greater size. Note further that each of these companies is selling something that is of little direct use to them. Neither has the sort of distribution network that would allow them to sell their products overseas.

These sorts of risk sharing arrangements are not limited to the pharmaceutical industry or even to for-profit firms. The Sisters of Mercy sought to reorient its system from serving the suburbs to serving the inner-city poor. To do so Mercy Health System built a new hospital in a poor area, which in turn created three problems: a massive bill for debt service, large losses on its new facility, and lack of management experience in serving this population. Mercy Health System addressed all three of these problems by entering into a joint venture with Henry Ford Health System. In exchange for an interest in two of Mercy's suburban facilities, Ford offered protection against up to $4 million in annual losses on Mercy's new hospital and a CEO with experience in serving the inner-city poor. This joint venture helped Mercy Health System better realize its goals, even though one of them was not profit-driven.

This example illustrates another facet of risk sharing: organizations often seek to share the enormous cost of acquiring a key competency. Working with a knowledgeable partner allows the organization to gain experience in an area. It takes a lot of time and money to build expertise, and joint ventures can reduce the risk of doing so. Of course the organization must assess what the gains are for the partner, who is also gaining expertise and profits.

The worldwide growth of selective contracting has changed healthcare management by increasing the risks that provider organizations must assume (Kirkman-Liff et al. 1997). In a pure fee-for-service environment, providers are at risk for costs per procedure that are too high. (And in a cost-plus environment, providers are not even fully at risk for excessive costs.) In a global pricing environment, in contrast, providers are at risk for variations in procedures per case as well as costs per procedure. In addition, the risks of global pricing can seem tame to providers who have signed capitation contracts. They are at risk for variations in cases per enrollee in addition to the other risks mentioned earlier.

To cope with these increased risks, providers have adopted a number of strategies. A major initiative has been to diversify their service offerings. This allows organizations to treat patients in appropriate least-cost settings, such as ambulatory surgery centers, skilled nursing units, and urgent care units. Lack of access to alternatives should not be the reason why patients are treated in high-cost settings. In addition, to improve management, healthcare organizations have increasingly invested in information systems. Without reliable information about service use and costs, providers can neither manage costs nor contract profitably with insurers.

With reliable information, providers have begun to change how care is delivered. This process, which is sometimes called the "industrialization" of healthcare, typically involves making clinical pathways and continuous quality improvement integral parts of the organization.

In many ways, the most important change has been the increasing integration of clinicians into management. Part of this integration entails developing clinical managers, physicians, and nurses with day-to-day management roles. Another part of this integration involves aligning the incentives of all the participants. Of course, for organizations that have accepted the risks of capitation, a good stop-loss insurance policy is usually a part of the strategy for managing increased risk.

4.8 Diversification

Diversification consists of identifying a portfolio of projects or therapies that are not highly, positively correlated. Figure 4.2 compares investing in a clinic, a trauma unit, and a 50 percent share of both. Return on investment forecasts for the projects depend on whether the growth of an HMO is rapid, moderate, or slow. The clinic is a better investment than the trauma unit (higher expected profits and lower standard deviation of profits). The portfolio is also a better investment than the trauma unit (higher expected profits and lower standard deviation of profits). The portfolio might be a better investment than the clinic for a risk averse investor (lower expected profits but a lower standard deviation of profits).

FIGURE 4.2
Diversification and
Risk Reduction

	HMO growth				
	Rapid	Moderate	Slow	Expected	Std. Dev.
Growth probabilities	0.160	0.700	0.140		
			Profits		
Clinic profits	10%	4.0%	−1%	4.3%	3.0%
Trauma unit profits	−3%	2.0%	13%	2.7%	4.5%
Portfolio profits (50% of each)	3.5%	3.0%	6.0%	3.5%	1.0%

4.9 Conclusion

The goal of describing, evaluating, and managing risk is to improve choices, not to identify perfect ones. Even when the evidence available to a decision maker is very good and a positive decision is made, bad outcomes can result. More often however, the information at hand falls far short of the ideal, prompting medical and managerial decisions that are made with inadequate information. For example, patients commonly must make therapeutic choices long before they know for sure what disease is causing their symptoms. Even in cases in which the disease has been positively identified, the consequences of the several treatment choices cannot be known with certainty.

Good management, however, can reduce risk and the consequences of risk. Some risks need not be taken if the payoff is not adequate. Some risks can be shared via joint ventures or insurance, or hedged with diversification. A balanced portfolio of projects and lines of business can be profitable in any market environment, while some risks can be ameliorated with good management. Reducing variations in costs (so that risks are lower in capitated environments) or reducing fixed costs (so that sales slumps do not hurt as much) can cut risk sharply. Then, of course, there is the old standby, which uses a high margin to reduce risk; if possible outcomes are a 15 or 11 percent return on equity, most managers will sleep well.

References

Cherney, A. 1996. *The Capitation & Risk Sharing Guidebook.* Chicago: Irwin.

Kirkman-Liff, B. L., R. Huijsman, T. Vander Grinten, and G. Brink. 1997. "Hospital Adaption to Risk-bearing: Managerial Implications of Changes in Purchaser-provider Contracting." *Health Policy* 39 (3): 207–23.

COST

Key Concepts

- Cost depends on perspective.
- Costs can be difficult to measure.
- Good management requires an accurate understanding of costs.
- The goods and services that an organization produces are called **outputs**.
- The goods or service that an organization uses in production are called **inputs**.
- **Incremental cost** equals the change in cost due to a change in output.
- **Average cost** equals the total cost of a process divided by the total output of a process.
- When large firms have a cost advantage there are **economies of scale**.
- When multiproduct firms have a cost advantage there are **economies of scope**.
- Higher quality should mean higher costs. If not, the organization is inefficient.
- Higher input prices mean higher costs.
- Costs depend on what is produced, technology, input prices, and efficiency.
- An **opportunity cost** is the value of a resource in its best alternative use.
- **Sunk costs**, which are any costs that you cannot change, should be ignored.

5.1 Understanding Costs

Understanding and managing costs are core tasks for managers. Whatever the mission of the organization, controlling costs must be a priority. This is especially true in healthcare, as increasing competition, growing excess capacity, and expanding risk-sharing make controlling costs more important than ever.

The low-cost producer of a good or service has an advantage. Pharmacies that can accurately dispense a product more cheaply and hospitals that can successfully carry out a therapy at a lower cost than the competition have long had, and continue to have, an advantage. The low-cost producer can win more contracts, enjoy higher profit margins, or more easily weather a slump. Until recently, a strategy was considered to be efficient if no other approach would yield the same outcomes with lower costs or if no other approach would yield better outcomes at the same cost. The bar has been raised, however. Capitation and case-based payment systems challenge us to think about health, not just medical care. Now efficiency means not just producing goods and services efficiently, but also producing health efficiently, which is more difficult.

In this chapter we will focus on what it takes to turn an organization into a low-cost producer. The starting point is to understand costs. While this might not seem difficult, we will need two definitions to describe costs. First, the goods or service that your organization uses in producing its outputs are called **inputs**. Second, **opportunity costs** equal the value of an input in its best alternative use. From this production-oriented perspective, then, costs simply equal the opportunity cost per unit of input multiplied by the volume of inputs that your organization uses. Reducing the *cost per unit* that your organization pays for inputs will reduce total costs, but real savings come from reducing the volume of inputs that your organization uses. To do this, managers must lead efforts to improve efficiency or make hard decisions to outsource production of goods and services if it makes the firm more competitive.

5.2 Cost Perspective

Despite its apparent simplicity, cost is a complex concept because of perspective and measurement difficulties. Cost depends on the perspective of the individual's position in the transaction. For example, a consumer will characterize the cost of a prescription in terms of his out-of-pocket spending plus any ancillary costs, such as the value of time spent to fill a prescription. A pharmacist will focus on her spending to obtain, store, and dispense the drug. An insurer will focus on its payments to the pharmacist for the prescription, plus spending for managing the claim. Each of these perspectives on costs is valid, and each is different.

Figure 5.1 details what costs look like from four perspectives. A pharmacist acquires a prescription drug for $10 and incurs $5 in processing, storing, and billing costs. The pharmacist should recognize that a reasonable return on her time and on her investment in the pharmacy represents the *opportunity cost*. (Both her time and her investment could be put to use in other ways. She is more apt to think in terms of requiring a mark-up over her explicit costs, but that works out to mean much the same thing.) The consumer is uninterested

FIGURE 5.1

Costs from Three Perspectives

	Cost of a prescription drug				Cost of a non-prescription drug			
	Pharmacy	Consumer	Insurer	Society	Pharmacy	Consumer	Insurer	Society
Wholesale price	$10	$0	$0	$10	$3	$0	$0	$3
Processing	3	0	0	3	1	0	0	1
Billing and payment	2	4	9	15	1	2	0	3
Return on assets	1	0	1	2	1	0	0	1
Retail price	(16)	5	11	0	(6)	6	0	0
Total	$0	$9	$21	$30	$0	$8	$0	$8

in the pharmacist's costs. What matters to him is his $5 copayment and the cost that he incurs when he drives to the pharmacy to pick up the prescription. Similarly, the insurer focuses on its share of the price plus its cost of paying the bill. Again, the insurer must factor in the *opportunity cost* of using its investment to provide pharmacy insurance benefits, but will probably express this in terms of a required return on investment. From the perspective of the insurer, having the patient use a non-prescription drug is quite advantageous. It avoids $21 in costs if it can switch the patient from the prescription medication. From the perspective of the consumer, the switch to the non-prescription medication saves very little. A small shift in costs might well make the consumer unhappy with the switch, even if the prescription and non-prescription medications were equally effective. Note also that costs look very different from the perspective of society than from the perspective of any of the participants when insurance plays a role. In contrast, when there is no insurance, the consumer's perspective on costs mirrors society's.

When discussing costs, if you do not clearly state a specific perspective, you will almost certainly arrive at the wrong cost. The part of cost that matters depends on your point of view. Your revenues are someone else's costs, and your costs are someone else's revenues. Failing to recognize this results in confusion.

Managers naturally want to focus on costs from the perspective of the organization in which they work. It should be stressed, however, that shifting costs to customers or suppliers seldom represents a good business strategy. Long-term business success rests on selling products that offer your customers excellent value and your suppliers adequate profits.

5.2.1 Measuring Costs

Cost can also be an elusive concept because important components of costs are difficult to measure—managers sometimes get confused when trying to calculate the opportunity cost of resources that have changed in value. For example, land that your organization purchased in the past may now be much more valuable if rents in the area have risen sharply, or much less valuable if rents have fallen. Most of the time, however, an input's opportunity cost is simply its market price.

A much more common problem arises when the link between the use of a resource and the organization's output is difficult to ascertain. For example, how much of the organization's information system does the intensive care unit "use" for each additional patient? While answering this type of question can be quite difficult, by focusing attention on **incremental costs** (the cost of the additional resources that you use when the output is slightly increased), economic models often radically simplify the process of understanding and managing costs.

These ambiguities pose a challenge, as managing costs is now more important than ever for healthcare organizations. The increasingly competitive environment forces organizations to reduce costs and to assess the profitability of activities. Both require a clear understanding of costs.

5.3 Average and Incremental Costs

To talk sensibly about costs we need to understand two very key concepts: *average cost* and *incremental cost*. **Average cost** equals the total cost of a process divided by the total output of a process. As seen in Figure 5.2, when total cost equals $6,600 and output equals 15, average cost equals $440. **Incremental cost** equals the change in the total cost of a process that is associated with a change in the total output of the process. (The terms *incremental cost* and *marginal cost* are interchangeable.) In this example, total cost rises from $6,000 to $6,600 as output rises from 10 to 15. So, incremental cost equals ($6,600 − $6,000)/(15 − 10), or $120.

In Figure 5.2, average cost is significantly larger than incremental cost. This is quite common and quite important. The difference is common because many processes require resources (like equipment or key personnel) that are difficult to change as output varies. For example, to start a pharmacy a pharmacist will have to rent a building and commit her own time. If sales fall short of expectations the rent will not change. Such a component of total cost is called a **fixed cost**. In contrast, some labor costs and the cost of restocking the pharmacy will vary with sales, and are **variable costs**. Average costs include both fixed and variable cost, but incremental costs include only variable costs. The fact that average costs often exceed incremental costs is important because management decisions often hinge on knowing how much it costs to increase or decrease production of a good or service. Your willingness to negotiate with an insurer who offers $300 per service is likely to depend on whether you believe that an additional service will cost you $440 or $120. Correctly understanding costs is crucial.

Both average and incremental cost are important concepts, although the main contribution of economists to decision making is their constant reminder to focus on incremental values. Most management decisions are incremental in nature. "Should we increase hours in the pediatric clinic?" or "Should we reduce evening pharmacy staff?" or "Should we accept patients needing skilled nursing care?" These sorts of decisions demand data on incremental costs.

In addition to being the most relevant for managers, incremental costs are much easier to calculate than average costs. Average cost calculations always involve difficult questions such as, "How much of the costs of the chief financial officer's office should we allocate to the pediatrics department?" In contrast, incremental cost calculations involve simpler calculations that most clinicians or front-line managers can do: "What additional resources will we need to keep the pediatric clinic open until 8 p.m. on Wednesdays and what are the opportunity costs of those resources?"

FIGURE 5.2

Average and Incremental Costs

Quantity	1	10	15
Total cost	$5,100	$6,000	$6,600
Average cost	$5,100	$600	$440 = 6600/15
Incremental cost		$100	$120 = (6600−6000)/(15−10)

To decide whether to start or stop a service, a manager needs to compare average revenue and average cost. For example, a telemedicine program that has average revenue of $84 and average cost of $98 is unprofitable. To decide whether to expand or contract, a manager must compare how revenue and costs will change, which makes information about incremental costs essential. Usually confusions about cost arise because one person is talking about average cost and another is talking about incremental cost (or because one person is talking about costs to society and the other is talking about costs to the organization). Clear thinking requires understanding the difference between these two concepts.

5.4 Factors That Influence Costs

Producer costs depend on what is produced (outputs), the prices of inputs, technology, and efficiency. We will explore each of these in turn.

5.4.1 Outputs

Differences in outputs can profoundly affect costs. Firms that produce large volumes of a good or service may have lower costs than firms that produce small volumes. When large firms have a cost advantage this is referred to as **economies of scale**. Firms that produce several different kinds of goods or services may have lower costs than firms that produce just one. The cost advantages multiproduct firms have are called **economies of scope**. Both economies of scale and scope result from sharing resources. For example, a large pharmacy may be able to use automated dispensing equipment that would not make sense for a small pharmacy. If the large pharmacy had lower costs per prescription dispensed as a result, it would be benefiting from economies of scale. Or, a nursing home that offers both skilled and intermediate care might find that its costs for intermediate care were lower than costs in homes that offered only intermediate care. This might occur because the cost of the director of nursing could be shared among all patients.

How much does arthroscopic knee surgery cost?

According to analysts for Valley View Hospital, who used a technique called *activity-based costing*, average costs total $942 in their hospital (Baker and Boyd 1997). Activity-based costing breaks surgeries down into activities (e.g., general operating room costs, use of the arthroscope itself, or intravenous set-up) and then assigns a cost to each activity by identifying the resources that it uses (e.g., scrub nurse time, equipment, and various types of overhead). The procedure cost is then calculated by multiplying the cost of each activity times the volume used.

This sort of information is vital for managing costs, strategic planning, and negotiating contracts. Managers who are not familiar with the healthcare field are usually shocked that few healthcare organizations really know what their costs are.

Few activity-based cost estimates calculate the incremental costs of procedures, which is information that managers need. It is clear, however, that Valley View's incremental cost of arthroscopic knee surgery is substantially less than its average cost. Their estimate includes allocations for fixed overhead and depreciation, neither of which really changes when volume changes.

Differences in the quality of outputs can affect costs as well. For an efficient firm, higher quality products cost more than lower quality products. Higher quality means that a good or service is more valuable in the eyes of the customer. If higher quality does not cost more, failing to provide it reflects inefficiency. In fact, healthcare's many opportunities to improve quality without increasing costs reflect just how inefficient most healthcare organizations are. Once an organization has become efficient, however, higher quality costs more. Better service, improved reliability, greater accuracy, less pain, and other enhancements usually increase costs.

5.4.2 Input Costs

Higher input prices mean higher costs. Only if a firm is inefficient or a perfect substitute for the higher-priced input is available will this not be true. An inefficient firm might be able to bring its costs down by shifting to a more efficient production process. For example, even if pharmacy technicians receive a pay increase, the cost of dispensing a prescription might not go up if the pharmacy switches to the more automated system that it should have been using before the wage increase. A firm can avoid higher costs by switching to a perfect substitute, although this is not likely. If, for example, an Internet access provider tried to raise its monthly rates, firms could switch to rival Internet access providers to avoid the cost increase.

More typically, however, higher input prices mean higher costs. A firm may limit the effects of a cost increase by changing its production process. When it does so, however, its costs will still rise somewhat. For example, a rise in electricity rates could be partially avoided by switching to more efficient lights, which would initially cost more to purchase and install.

5.4.3 Technology

Advances in technology always reduce the cost of an activity. But technology choices illustrate how difficult it can be to talk about costs. For example, if an automated laboratory system increased cost per analysis, it would be absurd to install it. But, the automated system's *lower costs per analysis* may dramatically increase physicians' requests for analyses, so lower costs per analysis do not guarantee that laboratory costs will go down. Indeed, this sort of technology-induced increase in overall costs is quite common. Managers need to understand that the apparent contradiction arises because the same word, "cost," is being used to describe the expense per procedure and total expense for a unit or total spending for a product.

5.4.4 Efficiency

Increases in efficiency always reduce the cost of an activity. Production of almost every healthcare good or service can be made more efficient. Unfortunately, few production processes in healthcare have been examined carefully, and most healthcare workers have little or no training in process improvement. Consequently, mistakes, delays, coordination failures, unwise input choices, and excess capacity are routine. Techniques for improving production (Total Quality Management, Continuous Quality Improvement, and Continuous Process Improvement) are just beginning to be applied in healthcare, so there is much to be done.

Although it may seem that everyone should be in favor of improving efficiency, that is not the case. Greater efficiency often means that fewer workers will be needed, so those whose jobs are in jeopardy may not want to help improve efficiency. Others have limited incentives to participate in efforts to improve efficiency. Physicians must participate in changing clinical processes, yet most have little to gain from doing so. The gains may accrue to the healthcare organization, but the reductions in billings will be a problem for a physician or other healthcare worker not employed by the organization. Devising incentives that will encourage workers and contractors to help improve efficiency represents a major challenge.

How large can the payoff from greater efficiency be?

The payoff can be quite large. Introduction of a clinical pathway for managing liver transplants reduced the cost per admission by over $8,000 in one hospital (Holtzman et al. 1998). A clinical pathway is a flow sheet that identifies when staff typically need to perform a duty and when patients can be expected to reach certain goals. Creation of a pathway usually increases efficiency because it encourages redesign of patient care and it improves management of care for individual patients. At the hospital in question, the average length of stay for liver transplants fell from 17.8 days to 11.8 days, and the complication rate fell from 57.1 percent to 18.5 percent. From these statistics, we can infer that the pre-pathway process of care was inefficient. When reductions in costs accompany improvements in the outcomes of care, it is obvious that the old system was inefficient. Since other care processes may be just as inefficient as this hospital's pre-pathway liver transplants, additional cost reductions or improvements in quality may be feasible.

5.5 Variable and Fixed Costs

Managing costs demands an understanding of opportunity costs and what might change costs. As stated earlier, an opportunity cost is the value of a resource in its best alternative use. Most of the time opportunity costs are easy to assess. The opportunity cost of using $220 in supplies is $220. The opportunity cost of using an hour of legal time that will be billed at $150 an hour is $150. Other cases demand more study. For example, the opportunity cost of a vacant wing of a hospital depends on what it might be used for. In a hospital with a census that may soon require reopening it, the opportunity cost of the wing will depend on its value as an acute care unit. In a hospital that needs a skilled nursing unit, its opportunity cost would be determined by the wing's value in that role.

Sunk costs should be ignored. A **sunk cost** is any cost that you cannot change. A computer's purchase price is a sunk cost, as is money spent to train employees to operate the computer. If it does not make sense to use the computer given current needs, do not worry about its initial cost. The opportunity cost of the computer will depend on its value in some other use (including its resale value).

Changes in any of the factors identified earlier will affect costs. Increases in input costs will increase costs. Improvements in technology will reduce costs per unit of output. For efficient organizations, improvements in quality will increase costs. Increases in efficiency will reduce costs.

In the long run, all costs are **variable**. Buildings and equipment can be changed or built. How work is done can be changed. Additional personnel can be hired. In the short run, some costs are **fixed**. An existing lease may not be negotiable, even if the building or equipment no longer suits your needs. As you might anticipate, you should not focus on fixed costs in the short run, since you cannot change them. In the short term, these are sunk costs.

When fixed costs are substantial, average costs typically fall as output increases. The fixed costs are being spread over a larger and larger volume of output, so average fixed costs fall. As long as average variable costs are stable, this drop in average fixed costs plus average variable costs. As Figure 5.3 illustrates, average fixed cost drops from $30 to $15 as output rises from 100 to 200. If variable costs rise quickly enough, average total costs may rise despite the fall in average fixed costs. In Figure 5.3, variable costs rise by $10,000 as output increases from 200 to 300. As a result, average total cost rises to $60 even though average fixed cost continues to fall.

Fixed and variable costs are important concepts for day-to-day management of healthcare organizations. For example, an advantage of growth is that fixed costs can be spread over a larger volume of output. The idea is that lower average fixed costs result in lower average total costs, so profit margins can be larger. As Figure 5.3 makes clear, it is vital to ensure that growth does not result in increases in average variable costs large enough to offset any reduction in average fixed costs. Otherwise, growth might be unprofitable.

Misclassification of costs can also result in odd incentives. It is not unusual, for example, to allocate fixed overhead costs on the basis of some measure of output. Doing so can make growth appear much less profitable than it is, as the overhead costs allocated to a unit increase as it grows. So that unit managers are not discouraged from expanding, allocated fixed costs should not vary with output.

Output	Total cost	Fixed cost	Average total cost	Average fixed cost	Average variable cost
0	$3,000	$3,000			
100	5,500	3,000	$55	$30	$25
200	8,000	3,000	40	15	25
300	18,000	3,000	18,000/300 = 60	3,000/300 = 10	15,000/300 = 50

FIGURE 5.3

Fixed and Variable Costs

Marginal Costs and Emergency Room Usage

While it would seem obvious that the marginal cost of seeing a patient who is not critically ill in the emergency room is much higher than the cost of seeing him or her in a physician's office, a study by Dr. Robert M. Williams suggests that this may not always be true (1996). He points out that the marginal cost of squeezing in an adolescent asthma patient for a 4:00 p.m. visit in a physician's office will be quite small, but the marginal cost of seeing the same patient at 4:00 a.m. in a physician's office is likely to be quite high. In comparison, the cost of seeing an additional patient at 4:00 a.m. in a fully-staffed emergency room may not be particularly high. Dr. Williams estimated that the marginal cost of a non-urgent visit to an emergency room was about $25, far less than the average cost ($62) or the average charge ($124) for such a visit. He also estimated that the marginal cost of an urgent visit was much higher (about $148).

This work illustrates that good management decisions are hard to make without reasonable estimates of costs. It also explains why increasing numbers of emergency rooms have set up urgent care centers. These urgent care centers use emergency room staff and equipment to serve patients with minor injuries and illnesses at prices well below the standard charge for an emergency room visit.

5.6 Conclusion

Managing costs has become vitally important in healthcare. The low-cost producer *always* has an advantage. And the increasingly competitive environment is forcing healthcare organizations to reduce costs and reassess product lines as they seek to identify least-cost production techniques and core goods and services. This pressure has intensified as purchasers of goods and services have come to realize that high costs do not guarantee high quality and that high quality does not always incur high cost. Healthcare organizations are seeking to adopt cost-reducing technology, substitute high-cost for low-cost production techniques, become prudent purchasers of goods and services, and rethink what they produce. These changes present significant challenges, with even more on the horizon. Increasingly, healthcare providers are being challenged to improve the health of target populations in ways that are cost effective. This is more difficult than simply producing healthcare products efficiently.

References

Baker, J., and G. Boyd. 1997. "Activity-Based Costing in the Operating Room at Valley View Hospital." *Journal of Health Care Finance* 24 (1): 1–9.

Holtzman, J., T. Bjerke, and R. Kane. 1998. "The Effects of Clinical Pathways for Renal Transplant on Patient Outcomes and Length of Stay." *Medical Care* 36 (6): 826–34.

Williams, R. M. 1996. "The Costs of Visits to Emergency Departments." *New England Journal of Medicine* 334 (10): 642–46.

6

THE DEMAND FOR HEALTHCARE PRODUCTS

Key Concepts

- The **quantity demanded** is the amount of a good or service purchased at a specific price when all other factors are held constant.
- Usually the quantity of a product that is demanded falls when its price rises.
- **Demand** (a demand curve) describes the amounts of a good or service that will be purchased at different prices when all other factors are held constant.
- **Market demand** is the sum of the demands of all consumers in a market.
- An **increase** or **decrease in demand** reflects a shift in the entire list of amounts purchased at different prices. An increase or decrease in demand results when one of the other factors that influences consumer decisions changes.
- Other factors that influence demand are consumer income, insurance coverage, perceptions of health status, perceptions of the productivity of goods and services, the prices of other goods and services, and tastes.
- The amount of money that a consumer directly pays for a good or service is called the **out-of-pocket price** of that good or service.
- Because of insurance, the total price and out-of-pocket price can be quite different.
- A **complement** is a good or service that is used in conjunction with another good or service. Demand for a good falls if a complement increases in price.
- A **substitute** is a good or service that is used instead of another good or service. Demand for a good rises if a substitute increases in price.

6.1 Introduction

Demand is one of the central ideas of economics, and it underpins many of the contributions of economics to public and private decision making. Demand is defined as the amount of a good or service that will be purchased at different prices when all other factors are held constant. Analyses of demand tell us that human wants are seldom absolute. More often they are conditioned by the questions, "Is the good or service really worth the cost? Is its value greater than that cost?" These questions are central to understanding healthcare economics.

6.1.1 Demand

As a very practical matter, demand forecasts are essential parts of management. Most managerial decisions are based on revenue projections, which in turn depend on estimating the volume of sales given the price that managers set. This estimate of volume, given a price, is one application of demand theory known as a *demand forecast.* The ability to understand the relationship between price and quantity must be a part of every manager's skill set. At a fundamental level, demand forecasts allow managers to decide whether to produce products at all and, if they do produce them, how much to charge. Suppose that you conclude that the direct cost of providing therapeutic massage is $48 and that you will need to charge at least $75 to cover other costs and offer an attractive profit margin. At a price of $75 will you have enough customers to make this a sensible addition to your product line? Demand analyses are designed to answer questions like this.

Using Demand Forecasts to Increase Profits

Longs Drug Stores uses demand forecasts to dramatically reduce its inventory costs (Doan 1999). Nonstop Solutions uses Longs' sales data to forecast sales patterns for each of its 362 retail stores. The Nonstop algorithm, based on research by its founder, Professor Hau Lee of Stanford University, considers factors such as the season and the demand trends for individual stores. It then translates these demand forecasts into inventory recommendations for each store for individual pharmaceuticals, dosages, and bottle sizes. Armed with this information, Longs Drug Stores was able to sharply reduce inventories at both its central warehouse and its stores. For example, it was able to reduce its inventory of Xanx, an antianxiety drug, from 26 days worth of orders to 6.7 days worth. This single change reduced the amount of cash devoted to inventory by $15,210.

In addition to increasing profits, the Nonstop system allows pharmacists to concentrate on serving customers rather than managing inventory. For example, no longer occupied with checking his inventory, one pharmacist was able to develop a program for in-store cholesterol screenings.

6.1.2 Market Systems

We, like every society, need to somehow ration goods and services (including medical). Human wants are nearly infinite, but our capacity to satisfy those wants is decidedly finite. As a result, we must develop a system for determining which wants will be satisfied and which wants will not. **Market systems** use price to ration goods and services, and doing so has some advantages. A price system costs relatively little to operate, is usually self-correcting (e.g., prices fall when the quantity supplied exceeds the quantity demanded), and allows individuals with different wants to make different choices. These are important advantages. The problem is that markets work by limiting the choices of some consumers. As a result, even if the market *process* is seen as fair, the market *outcome* may seem unfair. Wealthy societies such as ours, however, typically do not accept the exclusion of some consumers, perhaps because of low income or previous catastrophic medical expenses, from receiving valuable medical services.

The implications of demand are not limited to market-oriented systems, however. Demand theory predicts that if the use of care is not rationed by price, it will be rationed by other means, typically waiting times. Rationing methods that do not use price are often inconvenient for consumers. In addition, careful analyses of consumer utilization of services have convinced most analysts that medical goods and services should not be "free." Someone must pay, somehow, because modern healthcare requires the services of highly skilled professionals, complex and elaborate equipment, and specialized supplies. All of these resources could be used in other ways, meaning that the costs of healthcare are quite real. Even the resources used in care for which there is no charge represent a cost to someone. Were care truly costless for consumers, they would use it until it offered no additional value to them. Today this understanding is reflected in the public and private insurance plans of most nations.

6.1.3 Indirect Payments and Insurance

Because the burden of healthcare costs falls primarily on an unfortunate few, health insurance is common. Insurance creates another role for demand analyses. To design sensible insurance plans we need to understand the public's valuation of services. Insurance plans seek to identify benefits that the public is willing to pay for, albeit indirectly. The public may pay directly (**out-of-pocket**) or indirectly in the form of health insurance premiums, taxes, wage reductions, or higher prices for other products. Understanding what value the public places on services is especially important in the healthcare sector because indirect payments are so common. When consumers pay directly, valuation is not very important (except for making revenue forecasts). A consumer who refuses to buy a $7.50 bottle of aspirin from an airport vendor because it is "too expensive" is making a clear statement about value. In contrast, a Medicare patient who thinks that coronary artery bypass graft surgery is a good buy at a cost of $1,000 is not providing us with very useful information. The surgery costs more than $30,000, but the patient and taxpayers pay most of the bill indirectly. Because so much of medical care is purchased indirectly, with the assistance of public or private insurance, it is often difficult to assess whether the value of goods and services are as large as their costs.

6.2 Why Demand for Healthcare Is Complex

The demand for medical care is more complex than demand for many goods for four reasons:

1. The price of care often depends on insurance coverage. Insurance has powerful effects on demand and makes analysis more complex.
2. Healthcare decisions are typically quite perplexing, since consumers would prefer to be healthy and not need medical services. Such services are of value largely because of their effect on health. The links between medical care and health outcomes are often difficult to ascertain at the

population level (where the average effect of care is what matters) and are stunningly complex at the individual level (where "what happens to me" is what matters). Forced to make hard choices, consumers may make bad choices.

3. This complexity contributes to the lack of information that consumers have about costs and benefits of care. Such "rational ignorance" is quite natural, as many consumers will not have to make most healthcare choices, and it makes no sense to be prepared to do so.

4. The net effect of complexity and consumer ignorance is that producers have significant influence on demand. Quite naturally, consumers turn to healthcare professionals for advice. Unfortunately, because they are human, professionals are likely to make choices that reflect their own values and incentives as well as those of their patients.

By itself, demand is complicated. To keep things as simple as possible, we will begin by examining the demand for medical goods and services in a situation in which insurance and the guidance of healthcare professionals play no role (e.g., demand for over-the-counter pharmaceuticals, such as aspirin). We will then look at the effect of insurance on demand, keeping professional advice out of the discussion, using the demand for dental prophylaxis as our example. Finally, we will examine demand when provider advice is involved.

6.3 Demand Without Insurance and Healthcare Professionals

A consumer's decision to buy a particular good or service reflects a seemingly maddening array of considerations. For example, a consumer with a headache who considers buying a bottle of aspirin must factor in his perceptions of its benefit compared to his other choices. Those other choices might include taking a nap, going for a walk, taking another nonprescription analgesic, or consulting with a physician.

Economic models of demand radically simplify descriptions of consumer choices by stressing three key relationships:

1. the effect of changes in the price of a good or service;
2. changes in the prices of related goods or services; and
3. the effect of changes in consumers' incomes on the amount of goods and services they purchase.

This simplification of consumer choices is of immense value to firms and policy makers, who really cannot change much besides prices and incomes. What they must remember when using such a simple model, however, is the potential effect of public information campaigns (including advertising) on consumers' choices. Beliefs and perceptions about their health and available products can have powerful effects on the decisions consumers make.

6.3.1 Changes in Price

Analysts use statistical techniques to estimate how much the quantity demanded will change if the price of a product changes, if income changes, or if other factors change. The fundamental prediction of demand theory is that the quantity demanded will decrease when the price of a good or service rises. The quantity demanded may decrease because some consumers buy smaller amounts of a product (such as analgesics) or because a smaller proportion of the population chooses to buy a product (as might be the case with dental prophylaxis). Figure 6.1 illustrates this sort of relationship. On demand curve D_1 a price reduction from P_1 to P_2 increases the quantity demanded from Q_1 to Q_2.

Figure 6.1 also illustrates a shift in demand. At each price, demand curve D_2 indicates that the quantity demanded will be smaller than with demand curve D_1. Alternatively, at each volume, willingness to pay will be smaller with D_2. This sort of shift might be due to a drop in income or in the price of a substitute, an increase in the price of a complement, a change in demographics or consumer information, or other factors. (We will explore demand shifts and supply shifts in more detail in Chapter 9.)

Demand curves can also be interpreted as meaning that prices will have to be cut to increase the volume of sales. This might occur because consumers who are not willing to pay what the product now costs will enter the market at a lower price. It might also occur because current consumers may use more of the product at a lower price.

Demand curves do not have to be straight lines. Like Figure 6.1, Figure 6.2 also shows a shift in demand. In Figure 6.2, however, the demand curves are not straight lines.

Substitution explains why demand curves generally slope down (i.e., why consumption of a product usually falls if its price rises). **Substitutes** exist for most goods and services—products that could be used instead of the product itself.

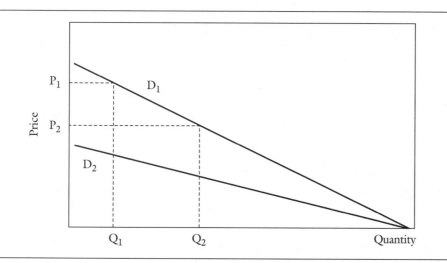

FIGURE 6.1
Linear Demand

FIGURE 6.2

Nonlinear Demand

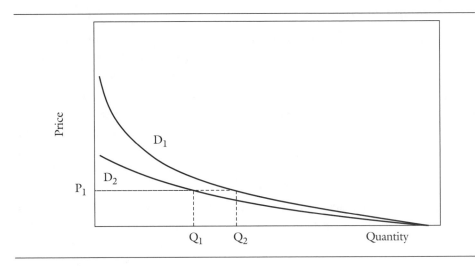

When the price of a product is high compared to the substitute, more people choose the substitute. For aspirin those substitutes included taking a nap, going for a walk, taking another nonprescription analgesic, or consulting with a physician. If "close" substitutes are available, changes in a product's price could lead to large changes in consumption. If none of the alternatives are "close" substitutes, changes in a product's price will lead to smaller changes in consumption. Taking another nonprescription analgesic is a close substitute for taking aspirin, so we would anticipate that consumers would be sensitive to changes in the price of aspirin.

Substitution is not the only effect of a change in price. When the price of a good or service falls, the consumer has more money to spend on all goods and services. Most of the time this "income effect" reinforces the "substitution effect," so we can predict with confidence that a price reduction will cause consumers to buy more of the good. In a few cases, things get murkier. A pay raise, for example, makes up for the income that you forego by working fewer hours. At first you might think that a higher wage would reduce the amount of time off you request. At the same time however, now that you have more income, you might actually want to take more time off for pleasure. In these cases, empirical work is necessary to predict the effect of a change in prices.

Two points about price sensitivity should be made here. First, a general perception that use of most goods and services will fall if prices rise is helpful. Second, managers need more precise guidance. How much will sales increase if prices are reduced by 10 percent? Will total revenue rise or fall as a result? Answering these questions requires empirical analysis. Fleshing out general notions about price sensitivity with estimates is one of the tasks of economic analysis, which uses agreed-upon terminology to talk about how much the quantity demanded will change in response to a change in income, the price of the product, or the prices of other products. Economists describe these relationships in terms of elasticities, which we will discuss later.

6.3.2 Factors Other than Price

Changes in factors other than the price of a product can shift the entire demand curve. Changes in beliefs about the productivity of a good or service, in consumer preferences, in the prices of related goods and services, and in income can shift the demand curve.

Beliefs about the health effects of products are obviously central to a discussion of the demand for health services. Few people want aspirin for its own sake. Like the demand for most medical goods and services, the demand for aspirin depends on consumers' expectations about its effects. These consumer expectations have two dimensions. The first depends on consumers' beliefs about health. If consumers believe that they are healthy, they are unlikely to purchase goods and services to improve their health. The second depends on consumers' beliefs about how much a product will improve health. If I have a headache, but do not believe that aspirin will offer relief, I will not be willing to spend money on it. Health status and beliefs about the capacity of goods and services to improve health underpin demand.

Demand is a useful construct only if consumer preferences remain stable enough to allow predictions of responses to changes in prices and incomes, and if changes in prices and incomes are important determinants of consumption decisions. If on Tuesday 14 percent of the population thinks that taking aspirin is something to be avoided (whether it works or not) and on Friday 24 percent of the population thinks this, demand models will be of little use. We would need to track changes in attitudes, not changes in prices. Alternatively, if routine advertising campaigns could easily change consumers' opinions about aspirin, tracking data on incomes and prices would be of little use. It appears that preferences usually are stable enough for demand studies to be useful, so managers can rely on them to make pricing and marketing decisions.

Changes in income and wealth usually result in changes in demand. In principle, an increase in income or wealth could shift the demand curve out (more consumption at every price) or in (less consumption at every price). In practice, increases in income or wealth usually shift out demand, as consumers with larger budgets buy more of most products.

Changes in the prices of related goods also shift demand curves. Related goods consist of substitutes and complements. **Substitutes** are products used instead of the product in question. For example, ibuprofen is a substitute for aspirin, and intravenous thrombolytic therapy is a substitute for angioplasty for patients with acute myocardial infarction. (A substitute need not be a perfect substitute, just an alternative in some cases.) **Complements** are products used in conjunction with the product in question. A reduction in the price of a substitute usually shifts the demand curve in (reduced willingness to pay at every volume). For example, if the price of ibuprofen fell, some consumers would be tempted to switch from aspirin to ibuprofen and the demand for aspirin would shift in. Conversely, an increase in the price of a substitute usually shifts the demand curve out (increased willingness to pay at every volume). For example, if the price of ibuprofen rose, some consumers would be tempted to switch from ibuprofen to aspirin and the demand for aspirin would shift out.

Consumers Choose Lower Prices

If given the opportunity to choose, will consumers choose less-expensive health insurance plans? Some evidence from California suggests that they will (Buchmueller and Feldstein 1997). In 1994 the University of California changed its benefits policy. Instead of basing its contribution on the average premium, the University limited its contribution to the cheapest policy available to all of its employees. As a result, employees had to pay the entire difference between the least expensive plan and the plan that they chose.

Employees who faced higher premiums were much more likely to switch to less expensive plans. Only 5 percent of those facing no premium increase changed plans. In contrast, 30 percent of those facing a $20 per month increase switched plans. Employees were more apt to switch to a plan with characteristics similar to the plan they were leaving. Older employees and employees who had been with a health plan for some time were less likely to switch, presumably because they had built relationships with physicians and other health professionals in their existing network. One group of employees did not have to change physicians when they switched to a cheaper plan, and 80 percent of them switched.

Because benefits were standardized across plans, employees had an easier time comparing the costs and benefits of alternative plans. As advocates of managed competition suggest, consumers appear to be willing to choose cheaper health plans when they can keep the savings. This is another instance in which managers can save money by aligning the incentives for employees and the organization.

6.4 The Effect of Insurance on Demand

Insurance changes demand by reducing the price of covered goods and services. For example, a consumer who has dental insurance will pay only $10 for a routine examination if her plan covers 80 percent of the cost, instead of the full $50. In most cases the volume of routine examinations will increase as a result (primarily because a higher proportion of the covered population will seek this form of preventive care). The response will not typically be "large." Most consumers will not change their decisions to seek care because prices have changed. But managers should recognize that consumers will respond to price changes caused by insurance. (We will develop tools for describing responses to price changes and review the evidence on this score in the next chapter.)

Figure 6.3 depicts standard responses to increases in insurance coverage. An increase in insurance (a higher share of the population covered or a higher

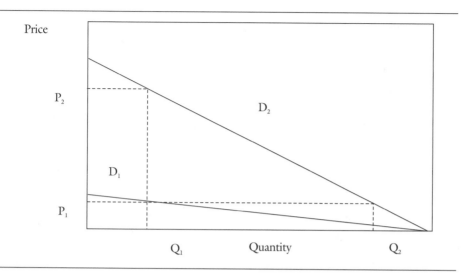

FIGURE 6.3
The Impact of
Insurance on
Demand

share of the bill covered) rotates the demand curve. Instead of D_1, the demand curve swings around to become D_2. As a result, the quantity demanded will rise from Q_1 to Q_2 if the price remains at P_1. Or, if the quantity were to remain at Q_1, the price could rise from P_1 to P_2.

For provider organizations, an increase in insurance coverage represents an opportunity to increase prices and margins. The rotation of D_2 has made it steeper, meaning that demand has become less sensitive to price. As demand becomes less sensitive to price, profit maximizing firms will seek higher margins (that margins have become higher means that the cost of production will represent a smaller share of what consumers pay for a product). Higher prices and increased quantity mean that expansion of traditional fee-for-service insurance will result in substantial increases in spending.

Increased Cost Sharing

Demand theory implies that having patients pay a larger share of the bill, usually called "increased cost-sharing," should reduce consumption of care. Does it? A landmark study by the Rand Corporation tells us that the answer is "Yes" (Manning et al. 1987). The Rand Health Insurance Experiment randomly assigned consumers to 15 different health plans in six locations and then tracked their use of care. Its fee-for-service sites had coinsurance rates of 0, 25, 50, and 95 percent. The health plans fully covered expenses above "stop-loss limits," which varied from 5 percent of income up to 15 percent. A **stop-loss** provision is the maximum amount that a consumer would have to pay out of pocket. As you can see, spending was substantially lower for consumers who shared in the cost of their care.

Increasing the coinsurance rate (the share of the bill that consumers pay) from 0 to 25 percent reduced total spending by nearly one-fifth. This reduction had minimal effects on health.

Coinsurance rate	Spending	Any use of care	Hospital admission
0%	$750	87%	10%
25%	$617	79%	8%
50%	$573	77%	7%
95%	$540	68%	8%

Costs were lower because consumers had fewer contacts with the healthcare system. The experiment went on for a number of years, and the suspicion that reducing use of care would increase spending later was not borne out. This study has been very influential. Based on the results of this study, virtually all insurance plans now incorporate some form of cost-sharing for care initiated by patients.

6.5 The Effect of Provider Advice on Demand

Consumers are often rationally ignorant about the healthcare system and the particular decisions that they need to make. They are ignorant because medical decisions are complex, they are unfamiliar with the options open to them, they lack the skills and information that they need to compare their options, and they lack time to make a considered judgment. This ignorance is rational because consumers do not know what choices they will have to make, because the cost of acquiring skills and information are high, and the benefits of acquiring these skills and information are unknown.

Consumers routinely deal with situations in which they are ignorant. Few consumers really know whether their car needs a new constant velocity joint, whether their roof should be replaced or repaired, or whether they should sell their stock in Cerner Corporation. Of course, consumers know that they are ignorant and respond to this by seeking to identify an **agent**, someone who is knowledgeable and will offer advice that advances their interests. Most people with medical problems choose a physician to be their agent.

Using an agent reduces, but does not eliminate, the problems associated with ignorance. Sometimes agents take advantage of **principals** (the consumers they represent) through out-and-out fraud (e.g., lying to sell a worthless insurance policy) or simple shirking (e.g., failing to check the accuracy of ads for a property). If consumers can identify poor performance on the part of an agent, fairly simple remedies can reduce the problems associated with consumer ignorance. In many cases an agent's reputation is of paramount importance, which instills a strong incentive to please principals. In other cases, simply delaying payment until a project has been successfully completed substantially reduces agency problems.

The most difficult problems arise when consumers have difficulty distinguishing bad outcomes from bad performance on the part of an agent. This is a fairly common problem. Did your house take a long time to sell because the market weakened unexpectedly or because your agent recommended that you set the price too high? Was your baby born via cesarean section to preserve her health or to preserve your physician's weekend plans? Most contracts with agents are designed to minimize these types of problems by aligning the interests of the principal and the agent. For example, real estate agents earn a share of a property's sale price, so that both the agent and the seller profit when the property is sold quickly at a high price. In similar fashion, earnings of mutual fund managers are commonly based on the total assets that they manage, so that both managers and investors profit when the value of the mutual fund increases.

Agency models have several implications for our understanding of demand. First, what consumers "demand" may depend on incentives for providers. Agency models suggest that changes in the amount paid to providers, in the way providers are paid, or in providers' profits may change their recommendations, and as a result change what consumers do. For example, consumers may respond to a lower price for generic drugs only if pharmacists have financial incentives to recommend them.

Second, provider incentives will have more effect on consumption of some goods and services than others. Almost by definition, provider recommendations will not affect patients' initial decisions to seek care. And, where standards of care are clear and generally accepted, providers will be less apt to change their recommendations when their incentives change. In these cases providers risk denial of payment, identification as a low-quality provider, or even malpractice suits.

Third, patients with chronic illnesses are often quite knowledgeable about the therapies that they prefer. When patients have firm preferences, agency is likely to have less effect on demand. In short, agency makes the demand for medical care more complex.

Most importantly, agency is one of the factors that makes managed care necessary. The other main factor is that insurance plans must protect consumers from virtually all of the costs of some very expensive procedures, so out-of-pocket costs need to fall to near zero. In the absence of asymmetric information, expenditures could usually be limited simply by changing consumer out-of-pocket payments. In many cases, however, provider incentives need to be aligned with consumer goals. (Of course, health plans also have an agency relationship with beneficiaries, and nothing guarantees that plans will be perfect agents.) Most of the features of managed care address the agency problem in one way or another. Global payments for services and capitation are designed to give physicians incentives to recommend no more care than is really necessary. Primary care gatekeepers are supposed to monitor recommendations for specialty services (from which they derive no financial benefit).

6.6 Conclusion

Demand is one of the central ideas of economics; therefore, managers must understand the basics of demand. In most cases, consumption of a product falls when its price is increased, and studies of healthcare products confirm this generalization. Understanding this relationship between price and quantity is a part of effective management. Without it, managers cannot predict sales, revenues, or profits.

To make accurate forecasts, managers also must be aware of the effects of factors that they do not control. Demand for their products will be higher when the price of complements is lower or the price of substitutes is higher. In most cases, demand for their products will be higher in areas with higher incomes. We will explore how to make forecasts in more detail in Chapter 7.

The demand for healthcare products is complex. Insurance and professional advice have significant effects on demand. Insurance means that there are three prices: the out-of-pocket price that the consumer pays, the price that the insurer pays, and the price that the provider charges. The quantity demanded will usually fall when out-of-pocket prices rise, but may not change when the other prices do. Because professional advice is important in consumers' healthcare decisions, the incentives that professionals face can influence consumption of some products. How and what professionals are paid can affect their recommendations, and recognition of this has helped spur the shift to managed care. To change patterns of consumption, managers may need to change incentives for both patients and providers.

References

Buchmueller, T., and P. Feldstein. 1997. "The Effect of Price on Switching among Health Plans." *Journal of Health Economics* 16 (2): 231–47.

Doan, A. 1999. "Vitamin Efficiency." *Forbes* 64 (11): 176–86.

Manning, W. G., A. Leibowitz, M. S. Marquis, J. P. Newhouse, N. Duan, and E. B. Keeler. 1987. "Health Insurance and the Demand for Medical Care: Evidence from a Randomized Experiment." *American Economic Review* 77 (3): 251–77.

7

ELASTICITIES

Key Concepts

- An **elasticity** is the percentage change in one variable that is associated with a one percent change in another.
- Economists use elasticities to avoid confusion about units.
- Elasticities are valuable tools for managers because they allow quick calculations of the effects of strategic choices.
- Managers can use elasticities to forecast sales.
- To avoid ambiguities, use arc elasticities, which use the average of the starting and ending values as the denominator of percentage change calculations.
- An **income elasticity of demand** is the percentage change in the quantity demanded that is associated with a one percent change in consumer income.
- A **price elasticity of demand** is the percentage change in the quantity demanded that is associated with a one percent change in the price of a product.
- A **cross-price elasticity** is the percentage change in the quantity demanded that is associated with a one percent change in the price of a substitute or complement.

7.1 Introduction

Elasticities are valuable tools for managers. Armed only with basic marketing data and reasonable estimates about elasticities, managers can make sales, revenue, and marginal revenue forecasts. In addition, elasticities are ideal for analyzing "what if?" questions. What will happen to revenues if we raise prices by two percent? What will happen to our sales if the price of a substitute drops by 3 percent?

Elasticities also reduce intentional and unintentional confusion in descriptions. For example, suppose that the price of a 500-tablet bottle of generic ibuprofen rose from $7.50 to $8.00. Someone who was seeking to downplay the size of this increase (or someone whose focus was on the cost per tablet) would say that the price rose from 1.5 cents to 1.6 cents per tablet. If you were experienced with such comparisons you would understand that describing this change in percentage terms eliminates any confusion about price per bottle or price per tablet. However, a potential source of confusion still exists: the change could be described as an increase of 6.67 percent (using the starting value of $7.50) or 6.25 percent (using the ending value of $8.00).

To avoid confusion in calculating percentages, economists recommend two courses of action. One is to be very explicit about the values used to calculate percentage changes. For example, one might say that the price increase to $8.00 represents a 6.67 percent increase from the starting value of $7.50. In our view, the best course of action is to use the average of the starting and ending values to calculate percentage changes to avoid complications that may confuse the unwary. For example, increasing the price by 6.67 percent and then cutting it by 6.25 percent returns the price right back to $7.50. Using the average price of $7.75 to calculate the percentages means that only one answer is possible: the price increased 6.45 percent.

7.2 Elasticities

An **elasticity** is the percentage change in one variable associated with a one percent change in another. For example, Newhouse and Phelps used statistical techniques to estimate that the income elasticity for physician visits was 0.04 (1976). The base for this estimate is average income, so this means that an income one percent above the average is associated with an average level of physician visits that is 0.04 percent above average. As we shall see, these apparently esoteric estimates can be quite valuable for managers.

First we need to learn a little more about elasticities. Economists routinely calculate three demand elasticities:

1. **income elasticity**: the percentage change in the quantity demanded that is associated with a one percent change in consumer income
2. **price elasticity**: the percentage change in quantity demanded that is associated with a one percent change in the price of a product
3. **cross-price elasticity**: the percentage change in the quantity demanded that is associated with a one percent change in the price of a substitute or complement

All can be represented as ratios of percentage changes. For example, the income elasticity of demand for visits would equal the ratio of the percentage change in visits (dQ/Q) that is associated with a given percentage change in income (dY/Y). (The mathematical terms dQ and dY identify small changes in consumption and income.) Therefore, the formula for an *income elasticity* would be $E_Y = (dQ/Q)/(dY/Y)$. The formula for a *price elasticity* would be $E_P = (dQ/Q)/(dP/P)$, and the formula for *cross-price elasticity* would be $E_R = (dQ/Q)/(dR/R)$, where R is the price of a related product.

Using the Newhouse and Phelps estimate of the income elasticity for physician visits implies that $0.04 = (dQ/Q)/(dY/Y)$. Suppose that we want to know how much higher than the average visits per person would be in an area in which the average income is 2 percent higher than average. As we are considering a case in which $dY/Y = 0.02$, we multiply this by both sides of the equation and find that visits should be 0.8 percent higher in an area with income 2 percent above the national average (0.02×0.04). From the perspective of a working manager, what matters is the conclusion that visits will only be slightly higher in the wealthier area.

7.2.1 Income Elasticities

Consumption of most healthcare products increases only slightly with income. As Figure 7.1 shows, consumption of healthcare products appears to increase more slowly than income. As a result, spending on healthcare will represent a smaller proportion of income among high-income consumers than among low-income consumers.

7.2.2 Price Elasticities

The price elasticity of demand is even more useful than the income elasticity of demand because prices depend on choices that managers make. Estimates of the price elasticity of demand will guide pricing and contracting decisions (as Chapter 9 will explore in more detail). Managers need to be careful in using the price elasticity of demand for three reasons. First, because the price elasticity of demand is almost always negative, a special vocabulary is necessary to describe the responsiveness of demand to price. It is very easy to get confused when talking about negative numbers. For example, -3.00 is a smaller number than -1.00, but -3.00 implies that demand is more responsive to changes in prices (a one percent rise in prices results in a three percent drop in sales rather than a one percent drop in sales). Second, changes in prices affect revenues both directly (via changes in price) and indirectly (via changes in quantity). Managers must keep this in mind when using the price elasticity of demand. Third, managers must be concerned with two very different price elasticities of demand: the overall price elasticity of demand and the price elasticity of demand for his or her firm's products.

Price elasticities of demand are usually negative. To avoid confusion, economists usually speak of demand as being *inelastic* or *elastic* (it is important to note that this terminology is not used when talking about other elasticities). When a one percent increase in price results in a less than one percent reduction in the quantity demanded, the price elasticity of demand will be between 0.00 and -1.00 and demand is said to be **inelastic**. When a one percent increase in price results in

Source	Date	Variable	Point estimate
Rosett and Huang	1973	Spending per person	0.25 to 0.45
Newhouse and Phelps	1976	Hospital admissions	0.02 to 0.04
		Physician visits	0.01 to 0.04

FIGURE 7.1

Selected Estimates of the Income Elasticity of Demand

Sources: Newhouse, J. P., and C. E. Phelps. 1976. "New Estimates of Price and Income Elasticities of Medical Care Services." Richard Rosett, ed. *The Role of Health Insurance in the Health Services Sector.* New York: Neal Watson.
Rosett, R. N., and L. Huang. 1973. "The Effect of Health Insurance on the Demand for Medical Care." *Journal of Political Economy* 81: 281–305.

a more than one percent reduction in the quantity demanded, the price elasticity of demand will be smaller than −1.00 and demand is said to be **elastic**.

It is important to recognize that inelastic demand does not mean that consumption will be unaffected by price changes. Suppose that, in forecasting the demand response to a 3 percent price cut, we use an elasticity of −0.20. Predicting that sales will drop by 0.6 percent, this elasticity implies that demand is inelastic but not unresponsive. Recall that a price elasticity of demand equals the ratio of the percentage change in quantity that is associated with a percentage change in price, or $(dQ/Q)/(dP/P)$. Using this formula and our elasticity estimate gives us $−0.20 = (dQ/Q)/ − 0.03$. After rearranging this and solving for the percentage change in quantity, we forecast that a 3 percent price cut will increase consumption by 0.6 percent, which is equal to $−0.20 \times −0.03$. Figure 7.2 shows that the demand for medical care is usually inelastic.

FIGURE 7.2
Selected Estimates of the Price Elasticity of Demand

Source	Date	Variable	Point estimate
Manning et al.	1987	Total spending	−0.17 to −0.22
Newhouse and Phelps	1976	Hospital admissions	−0.02 to −0.04
		Physician visits	−0.08

Sources: Manning, W. G., et al., 1987, Health Insurance and the Demand for Medical Care: Evidence from a Randomized Experiment, *American Economic Review* 77: 251–277.
Newhouse, J. P., and C. E. Phelps. 1976. "New Estimates of Price and Income Elasticities of Medical Care Services." R. Rosett, ed. *The Role of Health Insurance in the Health Services Sector.* New York: Neal Watson.

How elastic is the demand for ambulatory mental health services?

A number of studies have concluded that use of mental health services is more price sensitive than use of other ambulatory care. Analyses of ambulatory mental health services have found elasticities ranging from −0.44 to −1.00. This could be a statistical fluke resulting from adverse selection: consumers who anticipate using mental health services may choose insurance plans that offer generous coverage for such services. RAND Corporation researchers used data from the Health Insurance Experiment (which randomly assigned respondents to insurance plans) to resolve this issue (Keeler et al. 1988).

In fact, the RAND analysis, which is summarized in Figure 7.3, suggests that the demand for mental health services is more elastic than demand for general ambulatory medical services. Demand for each is inelastic, but consumers of mental health services appear to be much more price sensitive. Consumers facing a 25 percent coinsurance rate spent only 70 percent as much as consumers with no coinsurance requirement. Even though comparatively few consumers used any mental health services, this finding suggests that insurance plans that offer generous mental health benefits will cost more. In designing mental health benefits, managers will have to carefully weigh this.

Note that in calculating these elasticities, the RAND researchers used arc elasticities. This means that in calculating percentage changes, they used the average value as the base, calculating that a shift from 25 percent coinsurance to 50 percent coinsurance would represent a 67 percent increase $((50 - 25)/((50 + 25)/2))$.

FIGURE 7.3

Arc Elasticities of Demand for Mental Health and Medical Services[*]

Ambulatory mental health services	−0.79
Ambulatory medical services	−0.31

[*] The arc elasticity is computed over coinsurance rates ranging from 25 to 95 percent.
Source: Keeler, E. B., W. G. Manning, and K. B. Wells. 1988. "The Demand for Episodes of Mental Health Services." *Journal of Health Economics* 7 (4): 369–92.

7.3 Using Elasticities

Elasticities are useful forecasting tools. Armed with an estimate of the price elasticity of demand, a manager can quickly approximate the effect of a price cut on sales and revenues. As we noted earlier, however, managers need to use the correct elasticity. Most estimates of the overall price elasticity of demand fall between time price elasticities −0.10 and −0.40. For the market as a whole, the demand for healthcare products is typically inelastic. In contrast, demand is usually elastic for the products of individual healthcare organizations. Even though most healthcare products have few close substitutes, a product offered by one healthcare organization is usually a close substitute for the same product offered by another organization.

The price elasticity of demand faced by individual organizations typically depends on the overall price elasticity and the market share. Therefore, if the price elasticity of demand for hospital admissions is -0.17 and a hospital has a 12 percent share of the market, the hospital must anticipate that it faces a price elasticity of −0.17/0.12, or −1.42. This rule of thumb need not hold exactly, but there is good evidence that individual providers confront elastic demand. For example, Lee and Hadley estimate that the price elasticity of demand for the services of individual physicians ranged from −2.80 to −5.07 (1981). Indeed, as we will show in Chapter 8, profit-maximizing providers *should* set prices high enough so that demand for their products is elastic.

Armed with a reasonable estimate of the price elasticity of demand, we will now predict the effect of a 5 percent price cut on volume. If the price elasticity faced by a physician organization were −2.80, a 5 percent price cut should increase the number of visits by 14 percent, which is the product of −0.05 and −2.80. A prudent manager should recognize that his or her best guess about the price elasticity will not be exactly right and repeat the calculations with other values. For example, if the price elasticity is really −1.40, volume will increase by 7 percent. Or, if the price elasticity is really −4.20, volume will increase by 21 percent.

How much will revenues change if we cut prices by 5 percent and the price elasticity is −2.80? Obviously revenues will rise by less than volume because we have reduced prices. A reasonable estimate of the change in revenues is just the percentage change in prices plus the percentage change in volume. Prices will fall by 5 percent, quantity will rise by 7 to 21 percent, so revenues should rise by 2 to 16 percent. Our baseline estimate is that revenues will rise by 9 percent. If costs rise by less than this, profits will rise.

Elasticity of Demand and Waiting Time

One of the few determinants of demand that healthcare managers can control is waiting time. There is ample evidence that long waits discourage patients and drive up costs. One source estimated that the elasticity of demand with respect to waiting time was −0.958 in clinics, where waits tended to be long, and −0.252 in physicians' offices, where waits tended to be shorter (Acton 1975). This suggests that reducing waits by 10 percent could increase volume by 3 to 10 percent. In an environment in which many providers would like to add patients, reducing waits represents a strategy worth considering.

That reducing waits can sharply increase satisfaction with care is perhaps obvious. That higher satisfaction can lead to increased volumes or allow maintenance of higher prices may also be obvious. Long waits for patients often mean long waits for staff as well. One hospital reported that by changing procedures in its emergency department it was able to reduce the waiting time to see a physician by two-thirds. In the process, satisfaction scores nearly doubled and cost per visit fell by 12 percent, saving more that $422,000 (Anon. 1997). At the risk of belaboring the obvious, changes that increase satisfaction and reduce costs will generally improve a manager's career prospects.

7.4 Conclusion

An elasticity is the percentage change in one variable that is associated with a one percent change in another variable. Elasticities are simple, valuable tools that managers can use to forecast sales and revenues. Elasticities allow managers to apply the results of sophisticated economic studies to their organizations.

Three elasticities are common: income elasticities, price elasticities, and cross-price elasticities. Income elasticities measure how much demand varies with income; price elasticities measure how much demand varies with the price of the product itself; and cross-price elasticities measure how much demand varies with the prices of complements and substitutes. Of these, the price elasticity is the most important, because it guides pricing and contracting decisions.

Virtually all price elasticities of demand for healthcare products are negative, reflecting that higher prices generally reduce the quantity demanded. The overall demand for most healthcare products is inelastic, meaning that a one percent increase in a product's price results in a less than one percent reduction in the quantity sold. In most cases, however, the demand for an individual organization's products will be elastic, meaning that a one percent increase in a product's price results in a more than one percent reduction in the quantity sold. This difference reflects differences in how easily consumers can substitute one product for another. There are often few good substitutes for broadly defined healthcare products, so demand is inelastic. In contrast, the products of other healthcare providers are usually good substitutes for the products of a particular provider, so demand is elastic. Most of the decisions that managers make need to reflect that their organization's products face elastic demands.

References

Acton, J. P. 1975. "Nonmonetary Factors in the Demand for Medical Services: Some Empirical Evidence." *Journal of Political Economy* 83: 595–614.

Anonymous. 1997. "Cut Wages and Increase Revenue by Reducing Wait Times." *Health Care Cost Reengineering Report* 2 (5): 65–70.

Keeler, E. B., W. G. Manning, and K. B. Wells. 1988. "The Demand for Episodes of Mental Health Services." *Journal of Health Economics* 7 (4): 369–92.

Lee, R. H., and J. Hadley. 1981. "Physicians' Fees and Public Medical Care Programs." *Health Services Research* 16 (2): 185–203.

Manning, W. G., A. Leibowitz, M. S. Marquis, J. P. Newhouse, N. Duan, and E. B. Keeler. 1987. "Health Insurance and the Demand for Medical Care: Evidence from a Randomized Experiment." *American Economic Review* 77 (3): 251–77.

Newhouse, J. P., and C. E. Phelps. 1976. "New Estimates of Price and Income Elasticities of Medical Care Services." Richard Rosett, ed. *The Role of Health Insurance in the Health Services Sector.* New York: Neal Watson.

Rosett, R. N., and L. Huang. 1973. "The Effect of Health Insurance on the Demand for Medical Care." *Journal of Political Economy* 81: 281–305.

MAXIMIZING PROFITS

Key Concepts

- All healthcare managers should understand how to maximize profits.
- Most healthcare organizations are inefficient, so cost reductions can increase profits.
- To maximize profits, expand as long as marginal revenue exceeds marginal cost.
- **Marginal cost** is the change in total cost associated with a change in output.
- **Marginal revenue** is the change in total revenue associated with a change in output.
- Managers must understand their costs and not confuse incremental cost with average cost.
- Agency problems arise because the goals of stakeholders may not coincide.

8.1 Introduction

Substantial numbers of healthcare managers serve organizations that explicitly seek to maximize profits: for-profit hospitals, insurance firms, physician groups, and a broad range of other organizations. Even organizations that are not exclusively focused on the bottom line must balance their financial and organizational goals. Recognizing that "With no margin, there is no mission," many not-for-profit healthcare organizations operate like profit-maximizing firms as well.

As a result, even healthcare managers with objectives other than maximizing profits need to understand how to do so. A manager who does not understand the opportunity cost (in terms of foregone profits) of a strategic decision cannot lead effectively. Especially in today's market, as healthcare becomes more competitive, the differences between for-profit and not-for-profit firms seem likely to narrow.

Profits are the difference between total revenue and total cost. Maximizing profits requires identifying the product price (or quantity) and characteristics that maximize the difference between total revenue and total cost. To do this is fairly simple in principle, if complex in practice.

8.2 Cutting Costs to Increase Profits

The most obvious way to increase profits is to cut costs. This should be possible because most healthcare organizations are inefficient—they could produce the same output more cheaply or produce higher quality output for the same cost. This claim is supported by two types of evidence.

First is the common finding by quality management or reengineering teams that costs can be reduced with increased quality of care. The changes can be substantial. For example, the reengineering of a particular cardiovascular service at New York University Medical Center more than tripled the number of patients who were discharged in less than seven days and improved the quality of care, as evidenced by a lower readmission rate (Tunick et al. 1987).

Second, statistical studies paint much the same picture. For example, a sophisticated study of hospital efficiency concluded that inefficiency represented more than 13 percent of costs (Zuckerman et al. 1994). Opportunities to increase profits by increasing efficiency appear to be abundant.

As Figure 8.1 shows, the payoff from cost reductions can be substantial. The organization earns $40,000 on revenue of $2,400,000. This operating margin (profits/revenue) of 1.7 percent suggests that the organization is not particularly profitable. Reducing costs by only 2 percent changes this picture entirely. As long as the cost cuts represent more efficient operations, the cost reductions serve to increase profits by 118 percent.

8.2.1 Cost Reduction and Clinical Management

Increasingly, cost reductions require improvements in clinical management. This is true because differences in costs are primarily driven by differences in resource use, not differences in the cost per unit of resource. (Of course, an organization cannot maximize profits if it overpays for the resources that it uses.) In turn, differences in resource use are driven by differences in how clinical plans are designed and executed. At the very least, improvements in clinical management require the acquiescence of physicians, and, more typically, their active involvement. Even though many healthcare professionals make clinical decisions, physicians have a primary role in most settings.

Having recognized the importance of physicians in increasing efficiency, managers need to ask a basic question: Are the interests of the organization and its physicians aligned? That is, will changes that benefit the organization also benefit its physicians? If not, it would be naive to expect physicians to be enthusiastic participants in activities that may or may not benefit them, especially if the advantages for patients are not clear (or have not been made clear).

One fundamental responsibility of managers is to identify instances in which the interests of individual physicians are aligned with the organization, or change

FIGURE 8.1
Cost Reduction and
Increased Profits

	Status Quo	2% Cost Reduction
Quantity	24,000	24,000
Revenue	$2,400,000	$2,400,000
Cost	$2,360,000	$2,312,800
Profit	$40,000	$87,200

the environment so that they are. For example, physicians will generally benefit from changes in clinical processes that improve the quality of care or make it more attractive to patients. If presented in this fashion, physicians may understand its benefits for them. In other cases, however, it is unreasonable to expect physicians to participate actively in quality improvement activities without compensation. For independent physicians, explicit payments for participation may be needed. For employee physicians the same may be true, or participation may be a part of their contractual obligations. In neither case, however, can managers ignore the high opportunity cost of physicians' time spent away from clinical practice.

Where feasible, physician compensation can incorporate bonuses based on how well they meet or exceed clinical expectations. This has two advantages: it helps to align the incentives of the organization and its physicians and provides a continuing reminder to improve clinical management.

8.2.2 Reengineering and Quality Management

Reengineering and quality management are strategies for improving the performance of organizations from the perspective of their customers. Although reengineering stresses more radical changes and quality management stresses continuing incremental change, both share the premise that improvements in operations can increase profits.

The fact that reengineering and quality management initiatives *can* increase profits, however, does not mean that they will, or that doing so will be easy. Nothing guarantees that costs will fall, or that revenues will not fall faster than costs. These sorts of improvement initiatives often coincide with downsizing efforts, particularly in hospitals, which makes the staff wary (and can lead to the loss of the employees that the organization most wants to keep). Success under such circumstances requires skilled leadership.

A recent study of hospitals that started reengineering projects found that two years after the start of the projects, the typical hospital experienced modest improvements in profitability. A substantial number experienced very significant improvements, and a roughly equal number experienced significant deterioration (Serb 1998). Reengineering and quality management initiatives demand the time and attention of everyone in the organization, which often results in other things not getting done, or done less well. If not handled skillfully, reengineering and quality management initiatives can actually make things worse.

8.3 Profit Maximizing by Organizations

Organizations can also increase profits by expanding or contracting output. The basic rule for profit maximization in any business is "Expand as long as marginal revenue exceeds marginal cost. Contract as long as marginal cost exceeds marginal revenue," a logic that is quite straightforward. If increasing output increases revenue more than costs, or reducing output reduces costs more than revenue, profits rise as a result.

FIGURE 8.2

Marginal Revenue
and Marginal Cost

Quantity	Revenue	Cost	Profit	Marginal revenue	Marginal cost
100	$2,000	$1,500	$500		
120	2,400	1,600	800	$20	$5
140	2,660	1,840	820	13	12
160	2,880	2,120	760	11	14

What is marginal cost and marginal revenue (or incremental cost and incremental revenue)? **Marginal cost** is the change in total cost associated with a change in output. **Marginal revenue** is the change in total revenue associated with a change in output. The challenges lie in forecasting revenues and estimating costs.

As Figure 8.2 shows, increasing output from 100 to 120 increases profits, because the marginal revenue is greater than the marginal cost. Revenue increases from $2,000 to $2,400 as sales increase from 100 to 120 units, so marginal revenue equals $20 ($400/20). Costs increase from $1,500 to $1,600, so marginal cost equals $5 (100/20). The same is true for the expansion from 120 to 140. Marginal revenue falls because the organization cut prices to increase sales, and marginal cost rises because the organization is approaching capacity. Yet even though marginal revenue is nearly equal to marginal cost, profits still rise. Expanding from 140 to 160 reduces profits, however, and further price cuts push marginal revenue below marginal cost.

8.3.1 Incremental and Average Costs

Managers need to understand what their costs are and must be sure not to confuse incremental cost with average cost. Average costs may be higher or lower than incremental costs. As long as the organization is operating well below capacity, average costs will usually exceed incremental costs because of fixed costs. As an organization approaches capacity, however, incremental costs can rise quite quickly. If the organization needs to add personnel, acquire new equipment, or lease new offices to serve additional customers, incremental cost may well exceed average costs.

Why is it important to understand marginal costs and revenues?

A clinic is operating near its capacity when it is approached by a small preferred provider organization (PPO). The PPO wants to bring 100 additional patient visits to the clinic and pay $50 per visit for them. The manager eagerly accepts the deal, even though $50 is less than the clinic's average cost or average revenue. Shortly thereafter, another PPO approaches the clinic. It too wants to bring 100 additional patient visits to the clinic and pay $50 per visit. The manager turns them down. When criticized for this apparent inconsistency, the manager defends herself. "When the first PPO contacted us, we had excess capacity. Our marginal cost for those additional visits was only $10. Signing the first contract increased profits by $4,000, because our marginal revenue was $50 for those visits. When the second PPO contacted us, we no longer had excess capacity. We would have had to add staff to handle the additional visits. As a result, our marginal costs for the second would have been $510, and profits would have plummeted."

	Status quo	Adding the first PPO	Adding the second PPO
Quantity	24,000	24,100	24,200
Revenue	$2,400,000	$2,405,000	$2,410,000
Average revenue	$100.00	$99.79	$99.59
Marginal revenue		$50.00	$50.00
Cost	$2,040,000	$2,041,000	$2,092,000
Average cost	$85.00	$84.69	$86.45
Marginal cost		$10.00	$510.00
Profit	$360,000	$364,000	$318,000

Conceptually, the rules for profit maximization are quite simple. Expand as long as the return on investment is adequate and incremental revenue exceeds incremental cost. Cut back as long as the return on investment is adequate and incremental cost exceeds incremental revenue. Shut down if the return on investment is not adequate.

8.4 Return on Investment

When examining an entire organization, rather than a single well-defined project, most analysts focus on return on equity rather than return on investment. **Equity** is an organization's total assets minus outside claims on those assets. In other words, equity equals the initial investments of stakeholders (donors or investors) plus the organization's retained earnings.

What is an adequate return on investment? The answer to this question depends primarily on three factors: the yield on low-risk investments, the riskiness of the enterprise, and the objectives of the organization. All business investments entail some risk. Those risks may be high, as they are for a pharmaceutical company considering allocating research and development funds to a new drug, or those risks may be low, as they are for a primary care physician purchasing an established practice in a small town. In any case, those risks exist, and a profit-seeking investor will be reluctant to commit funds to a project that promises a rate of return similar to low-risk securities.

Consequently, when rates of return on low-risk investments are high, investors will demand high yields on higher-risk investments. The size of this risk premium will usually depend on a project's perceived risk. An investor may be content with the prospect of a 9 percent return on investment from a relatively low-risk enterprise, but will not find this adequate for an innovative, high-risk venture.

Because they must be responsive to the organization's stakeholders, managers must also avoid high-risk investments that do not offer at least a chance of high returns. What constitutes a high rate of return depends on the goals of the organization and the non-financial attributes of the investment. In some cases, an organization that is genuinely committed to nonprofit objectives will be willing to accept a low return (or even a negative return) on a project that furthers its goals. In short, the definition of an adequate return on investment will vary from organization to organization, but managers must understand how their organization defines an adequate return on investment if they are to understand their mission.

What sorts of rates of return do healthcare firms earn?

The answer to this question depends on the sector and the firm, but analyses by Cleverly (1997) show that hospitals' return on equity has risen slightly in recent years, from an average of 7.2 percent between 1992 and 1994, to 8.5 percent in 1995 and 1996. Managed care appeared not to affect return on equity very much, as returns were comparable in areas with both high and low managed care penetration.

8.5 Producing to Stock or to Order

Organizations can produce to stock or to order. Those that **produce to stock** make a forecast of demand and cost and produce output that is then stored in inventory. Medical supply manufacturers exemplify this sort of organization. More common in the healthcare sector, however, are firms that **produce to order**. They do the same demand and cost forecasts, but they do not actually produce anything. Instead, they set prices that are designed to maximize profits and then wait to see how many customers they get. Hospitals and physician practices are examples of organizations that produce to order. We make this point because discussions of profit maximization are usually framed in terms of choosing quantities or choosing prices, and someone learning about profit maximization may not understand that the logic is the same in both cases.

Therefore, while the discussion above has been largely framed in terms of firms that produce to stock, its implications apply directly to healthcare organizations that produce to order. These firms set prices based on their expectations about demand and cost. Only then do they discover whether they have set prices too high or too low. Prices have been set too high if marginal revenue is greater than marginal cost. The organization has given up the opportunity to make profitable sales. Prices have been set too low if marginal revenue is less than marginal cost. The organization has made sales on which the added revenue was smaller than the added cost. Organizations that produce to order must also make the same decisions about rates of return on equity. Is the 5 percent return on investment large enough to justify operating an organ transplant unit? How important is the unit to the organization's educational goals? What are the alternatives?

When organizations contract with insurers or employers, estimates of marginal revenue should be easy to develop. Simply calculate projected revenue under the new contract, subtract revenue under the old contract, and divide by the change in volume. For sales to the general public, economics gives managers a tool. It turns out that marginal revenue $= P(1 + 1/\varepsilon$, where P is the product price and ε is the price elasticity of demand. Most healthcare organizations face price elasticities in the range of 3.00 to 6.00, so marginal revenue can be much less than price. For example, if a product sells for \$1,000 and the price elasticity of demand is -1.50, its marginal revenue will equal \$1,000 $\times$ $(1 - 1/1.50)$, or \$333.33. In contrast, if the price elasticity of demand is -6.00, its marginal revenue will equal \$1,000 $\times$ $(1 - 1/6.00)$, or \$833.33. As you can see, as demand becomes more elastic, marginal revenue and price become more alike. Unless the elasticity becomes infinite, however, marginal revenue will be less than price.

What costs can we afford to incur, given the prices achievable in the market, and still earn a profit?

This, according to Shahram Heshmat, is the way that healthcare managers should approach decisions in a competitive marketplace (1997). From this perspective, managers should focus on incremental costs. These incremental costs may include incremental capital spending if the pricing decision results in an expansion that requires additional equipment, as well as more labor and materials. Costs that have already been incurred (e.g., depreciation on existing equipment) or would be incurred in any event (e.g., the salary of the unit manager) are not incremental costs, and should be ignored. Heshmat notes that a hospital might price a proposal to an HMO to add 150 additional normal births per month quite differently from a proposal to add 100 normal births per month. If increasing deliveries by 150 required adding staff and equipment and increasing deliveries by 100 did not, incremental costs would be much higher for the first proposal. A common mistake is to focus exclusively on average costs, which results in demanding prices that are too high. Heshmat closes by noting that efforts to build sunk costs into prices are shortsighted. It may justify past mistakes, but it misses opportunities to capture profitable volume.

8.6 Not-for-Profit Organizations

The strategies of not-for-profit organizations may differ from those of for-profit organizations because of an *agency problem* more severe than in for-profit firms, *differences in goals* because of not-for-profit status, and *differences in costs* because of not-for-profit status. These three forces have quite different effects on profits, so it is far from clear how much ownership matters.

8.6.1 Agency Problems

All organizations have an agency problem because the goals of managers may not coincide with the goals of stakeholders. For example, a higher salary clearly benefits a manager, but only benefits stakeholders in her organization if it enhances performance or keeps her from leaving (and a comparable replacement could not be attracted for less). This and other agency problems are part of every organization, yet not-for-profit organizations face three added challenges. First, they cannot turn managers into owners by requiring them to own company stock (which helps to align the interests of managers and other owners). Second, no one really "owns" the firm, so no one may be monitoring the managers to be sure that they are doing a good job for stakeholders. Finally, assessing the performance of managers in not-for-profit organizations represents a real challenge. If a not-for-profit organization earns less than a for-profit competitor, is it because of its focus on other goals, because of incompetence on the part of management, or because the firm's managers are using the firm's resources to live well? It is often difficult to determine.

What stakeholders do hospital managers have to satisfy?

A study of hospital executives identified the five most powerful groups of stakeholders: the hospital clinical staff, patients, the hospital management staff, the hospital professional staff, and the board of trustees (Fottler 1989). It should come as no surprise to learn that the goals of these groups were not identical. Physicians and nurses tended to focus on clinical quality and the adequacy of support services. Boards of trustees, while in favor of high clinical quality and adequate support services, tended to focus more on the bottom line. Disagreements among stakeholders can either give CEOs considerable flexibility or more problems.

8.6.2 Differences in Goals

While it may not do so, having goals other than profits can influence a firm's behavior. We can think of a not-for-profit firm as gaining benefits from pursuit of goals other than financial. In making decisions, the managers must consider how they affect the benefits derived from these other goals. To best realize the not-for-profit organization's goals, it should seek to equate MR + MB to MC (marginal revenue + marginal benefit to marginal cost). MB refers to the net marginal benefit to the firm from expanding a line of business. Three cases are possible:

1. If MB > 0, the not-for-profit will produce more than for-profit.
2. If MB = 0, the not-for-profit will produce as much as for-profit.
3. If MB < 0, the not-for-profit will produce less than for-profit.

A further complication is that MB may depend on other income. A struggling not-for-profit may act like for-profit, but a highly profitable not-for-profit may act quite differently.

8.6.3 Differences in Costs

Some reasons to believe that costs may differ for not-for-profit firms exist as well. First, the not-for-profit may not have to pay taxes (especially property taxes). This can make the not-for-profit firm's marginal costs lower. On the other hand, the not-for-profit organization's greater agency problems may result in greater inefficiency, and higher marginal costs.

The fundamental problem is that we cannot predict how not-for-profit firms will differ from for-profit firms. This is frustrating for analysts. It also raises a question for policy makers. If the community benefits of granting not-for-profit status are not clear and not guaranteed, why are not-for-profit firms being given a tax break? This is a natural question for policy makers to ask, so managers need to be ready with a convincing response.

Are not-for-profit hospitals really different from for-profit hospitals?

The research literature reaches no definitive conclusions on this question, but the Board of Assessors of Lebanon, New Hampshire, reached their own conclusion (Hallam 1998). They voted to end Dartmouth-Hitchcock Medical Center's exemption from local property taxes. This would make the center Lebanon's largest taxpayer, liable for $6 million in annual property taxes. Attorneys for the board claimed that Dartmouth-Hitchcock is a taxable organization under state law because it acts more like a for-profit company than a charity. The attorneys argued, for example, that the center "has purchased a number of for-profit physician group practices with no apparent change in operation of those practices."

Most hospitals are profitable, no matter who owns them. Indeed, in many respects not-for-profit and for-profit hospitals look very similar (Sloan 1998). On average, not-for-profit and for-profit hospitals provide similar amounts of uncompensated care, achieve similar levels of quality, and acquire new technology at about the same pace. Conversion to for-profit status, moreover, appears to change hospitals very little. The clearest difference between for-profit and not-for-profit hospitals seems to be that for-profit hospitals are less likely to be located in poor areas. In general, however, the differences between well-managed and poorly-managed hospitals are much larger than the differences between not-for-profit and for-profit hospitals.

8.7 Conclusion

Even managers of true not-for-profit organizations need to know how to maximize profits. Doing so entails identifying product lines that yield adequate returns on investment, pricing and promoting those product lines to allow realization of an adequate return on investment, and producing those product lines efficiently. Most healthcare organizations are less profitable than they could be because they are less efficient than they should be. It is important to recognize that increasing efficiency demands effective leadership. Cost reductions and quality improvements are easier to talk about than realize, especially since greater efficiency usually entails changing clinical plans (i.e., how physicians practice). Decisions to expand or contract need to be based on incremental costs and revenues. Few healthcare managers really know what their costs are, which presents a challenge.

Not-for-profit organizations may or may not be much different from for-profit organizations. In some cases their goals and performance are similar. Managers need to understand why the goals of not-for-profit organizations are worthy of tax preferences and be able to make that case to donors and regulators.

References

Cleverly, W. O. 1997. *The 1997–98 Almanac of Hospital Financial & Operating Indicators.* Columbus, Ohio: The Center for Healthcare Industry Performance Studies, 38.

Fottler, M. 1989. "Assessing Key Stakeholders: Who Matters to Hospitals And Why?" *Hospital & Health Services Administration* 34 (4): 525–46.

Hallam, K. 1998. "Taxed in New Hampshire: Study Says Academic Medical Center Acts Like For-Profit." *Modern Healthcare* April 6, 28.

Heshmat, S. 1997. Managed Care and the Relevant Costs for Pricing." *Health Care Management Review* 22 (1): 82–85.

Serb, C. 1998. "Is Remaking the Hospital Making Money?" *Hospitals and Health Networks* 72 (14): 32–33.

Sloan, F. A. 1998. "Commercialism in Nonprofit Hospitals." *Journal of Policy Analysis and Management* 17 (2): 234–52.

Tunick, P. A., S. Etkin, A. Horrocks, G. Jeglinski, J. Kelly, and P. Sutton. 1997. "Reengineering a Cardiovascular Surgery Service." *The Joint Commission Journal on Quality Improvement* 23: 203–16.

Zuckerman, S., J. Hadley, and L. Iezzoni. 1994. "Measuring Hospital Efficiency with Frontier Cost Functions." *Journal of Health Economics* 13 (3): 255–80.

SUPPLY AND DEMAND ANALYSIS

Key Concepts

- A **supply curve** describes how much producers are willing to sell at each price.
- A **demand curve** describes how much consumers are willing to buy at each price, or how much consumers are willing to pay at each quantity.
- At an **equilibrium price**, producers want to sell the amount that consumers want to buy.
- Markets generally move toward equilibrium outcomes.
- Expansion of insurance usually makes the equilibrium price and quantity rise.
- Insurance and professional advice influences the demand for medical goods and services.
- Regulation and technology influence the supply of medical goods and services.
- A demand or supply curve shifts when a factor other than the product price changes.

9.1 Introduction

Like the weather, healthcare markets are in a constant state of flux. Prices and volumes rise and fall. New products succeed at first, only to later fail. Familiar products falter and revive. Economics teaches us that, underneath the seemingly random fluctuations of healthcare markets, systematic patterns can be detected. Understanding these systematic patterns requires an understanding of supply and demand. Even though healthcare managers need to focus on the details of day-to-day operations, they also need an appreciation of the overview that supply and demand analysis can give them.

This chapter introduces and applies the basics of supply and demand, which illustrate the usefulness of economics. Even with very little data, managers can forecast the effects of changes in policy or demographics using a supply and demand analysis. For example, one can analyze the effects of added taxes on hospitals' prices, of increased insurance coverage on the output mix of physicians, or of higher electricity costs on pharmacies' prices. Supply and demand analysis is a powerful tool that managers can use to make both broad strategic and detailed pricing decisions.

9.1.1 Supply and Demand Curves

Figure 9.1 depicts a basic supply and demand diagram. The vertical axis shows the price of the good or service. In this simple case the price that sellers get is the same price that buyers pay. (When insurance or taxes come into play things get more complicated, as the price paid by the buyer is different from the price received by the seller.) The horizontal axis shows the quantity bought by customers and sold by producers.

The supply curve (labeled S) describes how much producers are willing to sell at each price. From another perspective, it describes what the price must be to induce producers to be willing to sell different quantities. The supply curve in Figure 9.1 slopes up, as do most supply curves. This upward slope means that, when the price is higher, producers are willing to sell more of a good or service or that more producers are willing to sell a good or service. This is true for two reasons. First, when the price is higher, individual producers are more willing to add workers, equipment, and other resources to sell more. In addition, higher prices allow firms to enter this market that could not do so at lower prices.

The demand curve (labeled D) describes how much consumers are willing to buy at each price. From another perspective, it describes how much the marginal consumer (the one who would not make a purchase at a higher price) is willing to pay at different levels of output. The demand curve in Figure 9.1 slopes down, meaning that, to sell more of a product, its price must be cut. A sales increase might be due to an increase in the share of the population that buys a good or service, an increase in consumption per purchaser, or some mix of the two.

The demand and supply curves intersect at the equilibrium price and quantity. At an **equilibrium price** the amount that producers want to sell equals the amount that consumers want to buy. In Figure 9.1, consumers want to buy 60 units and producers want to sell 60 units when the price is $100. This is an *equilibrium point*.

Markets tend to move toward equilibrium points. If the price is above the equilibrium price, producers' sales forecasts will not be met. In such cases, producers sometimes cut prices to sell more, or cut back on production. Either

FIGURE 9.1
Equilibrium

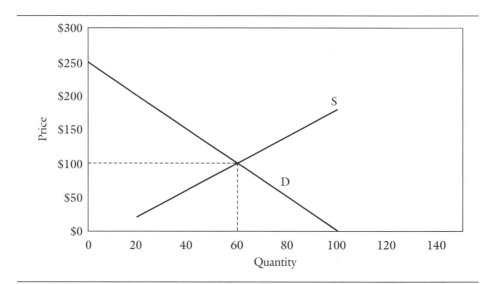

strategy tends to equate supply and demand. Alternatively, if the price is below the equilibrium price, consumers will quickly buy up the available stock. To meet this shortage, producers may raise prices or produce more, again equating supply and demand.

Markets will not always be in equilibrium, especially if conditions change quickly, but the incentive to move toward equilibrium is strong. Typically producers can change prices faster than they can increase or decrease production. A high price today does not mean a high price tomorrow, as prices usually fall as additional capacity becomes available. And a low price today does not mean a low price tomorrow, since prices are likely to rise as capacity gets reduced. We will explore this in more detail in our examination of the effects of managed care on the incomes of primary care physicians.

9.1.2 Provider Influence and Imperfect Competition

We offer two notes of caution. The first is that healthcare markets are complex. The influence of professional advice on consumer choices is a complication that is of particular concern. It may be misleading to assume that changes in supply will not spill over into consumers' choices (i.e., demand). If changes in factors that should not affect consumers' choices (such as providers' financial arrangements with insurers) influence providers' recommendations, a supply and demand analysis that does not take account of this effect could be quite misleading.

Second, and perhaps of even more importance, is that few healthcare markets fit the model of a competitive market (many competitors who perceive that they have little influence on the market price). We must condition any analysis on the judgment that healthcare markets are competitive enough to make conventional supply curves useful guides. In markets that are not competitive enough, producers' responses to changes in market conditions are likely to be more complex than supply curves suggest. This chapter will focus on applications of demand and supply analysis in which neither providers' influence on demand nor imperfect competition are likely to be problems.

9.2 Demand and Supply Shifts

We term a movement along a demand curve a *change in the quantity demanded*. Therefore, a movement along a demand curve simply traces the link between the price that consumers are willing to pay and the quantity that they demand. Demand and supply analysis is most useful to managers, however, in understanding how the equilibrium price and quantity will change in response to shifts in demand or supply. With relatively limited information, a working manager can sketch the impact of a change in policy on the markets of most concern.

What factors might cause the demand curve to shift to the right (for more to be demanded at every price or higher prices to be offered at every quantity)? We need detailed empirical work to verify the responses of demand to market conditions, but the standard list is quite short. Typically a shift to the right would result from an increase in income, an increase in the price of a **substitute** (a good or service used instead of a product), a decrease in the price of a **complement** (a good or service used with a product), or a change in consumer preferences.

Economists often use mathematical notation to describe demand. One example is $Q = D(P,Y)$, which says that the quantity demanded varies with prices, P, and income, Y. This means that quantity, the relevant prices, and income are systematically related. A demand curve simply traces out this relationship when income and all prices other than the price of the product itself do not change.

What factors might cause the supply curve to shift to the right (for more to be supplied at every price or lower prices to be sought at every quantity)? Typically a shift to the right would result from a reduction in the price of an input, an improvement in technology, or an easing of regulations. In mathematical notation we can write this $Q = S(P,W)$, where W represents the prices of inputs (the factors like labor, land, equipment, buildings, and supplies that a business uses to produce its product). Note, however, that while regulation is very extensive and technological change is rapid in the medical care sector, we do not make their roles explicit, unless they are the actual focus of an analysis.

Higher Pay Increases Physicians' Hours

Empirical analyses of supply find that higher pay results in higher volume (i.e., supply curves slope up). A study of young, male, self-employed physicians found that they fit this pattern (Rizzo and Blumenthal 1994). A one percent increase in hourly earnings increased annual practice hours by 0.23 percent. One reason for the muted response is that an increase in hourly earnings also increases total income, which usually leads to a reduction in hours. Confirming this expectation, the study found that a one percent increase in income from all sources reduced annual hours by 0.26 percent. Another factor is that many young physicians have spouses with high earning potential, which tends to reduce hours as well. A one percent increase in the spouse's income reduced annual hours by 0.02 percent. Change in either non-practice income or in a spouse's earning potential shifts the supply curve, illustrating that both practice and non-practice earnings affect annual hours of work. As is usually the case in labor supply analyses, both effects were relatively inelastic.

The implication for managers? That the way to get people to supply what you want is to pay them. Paying for visits will increase visits. Paying for quality will increase quality. This appears to apply to high-income and low-income workers alike.

9.2.1 An Expansion of Insurance

We begin our demand and supply analyses by looking at a classical problem in health economics: What will happen to the equilibrium price and quantity of a product used by consumers if insurance expands (i.e., either the insurance plan agrees to pay a larger share of the bill, or the proportion of the population with insurance rises)? This sort of change in insurance causes a **shift in demand,** as seen in Figure 9.2 This shift, or rotation, will take place any time the share of the total bill paid by insurance rises. An increase in the proportion of the population with insurance, a reduction in deductibles, or an increase in the share paid by insurance will have the same effect. As a result of this expansion of insurance, the equilibrium price rises from P_1 to P_2 and the equilibrium quantity rises from Q_1 to Q_2. While this description of the impact of insurance on healthcare markets may seem unrealistic, precisely this sort of scenario has been playing out in the market for prescription pharmaceuticals. As coverage for pharmaceuticals has become a part of more and more Americans' insurance, prices and sales of prescription pharmaceuticals have risen.

9.2.2 Influences of Regulation and Technology

Figure 9.3 depicts a shift in supply. The supply curve has contracted from S_1 to S_2. This shift means that at every price producers want to supply a smaller volume. Alternatively, it means that to produce each volume producers require a higher price. A change in regulations might occasion such a shift that made providing care more expensive. For example, suppose that state regulations mandated improved care planning and record keeping for nursing homes. Some nursing homes might close down, and the majority would raise prices to private-pay patients to cover the increased cost of care. The net effect would be an increase in the equilibrium price from P_1 to P_2 and a reduction in the equilibrium quantity from Q_1 to Q_2. A manager should be able to forecast this with no information other than the realization that the demand for nursing home care is not very elastic (meaning

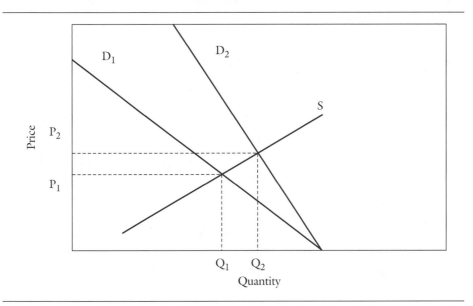

FIGURE 9.2

An Expansion of Insurance

FIGURE 9.3

A Supply Shift

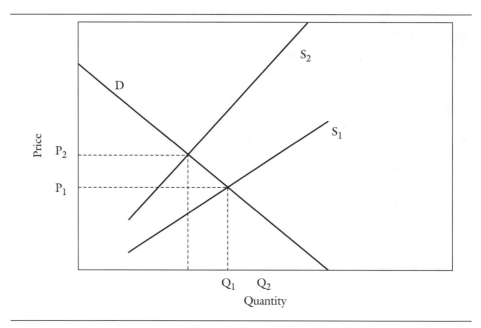

that the slope of the demand curve is steep) and that the regulation would shift the supply curve inward.

A final point about supply and demand needs to be emphasized: Responses to changing market conditions depend on how much time passes. A change in technology, such as the development of a new surgical technique, will not change supply very much initially. Over time, however, as more surgeons become familiar with the technique, its impact on supply will grow. Short-term supply and demand curves generally look very different from long-term supply and demand curves. The more time that they have to respond, the more the behavior of consumers and producers changes.

9.2.3 Increased Demand for Primary Care

The expansion of managed care during the early 1990s increased the demand for the services of primary care physicians, such as family practitioners and pediatricians (Simon, Dranove, and White 1998). During this period, managed care plans increased use of primary care gatekeepers to reduce use of specialists, and created a variety of incentives for (relatively low-cost) primary care physicians to meet more of the needs of plans' beneficiaries. Figure 9.4 illustrates the effects of this change. In the short run, the incomes of primary care physicians rose from I_0 to I_1 after demand shifted from D_0 to D_1. The supply of services from board certified or board eligible primary care physicians was relatively inelastic in the short run, as the slope of S_0 indicates. While some physicians could defer retirement or the shift into management, most of the supply response in the short run was due to more work by the existing cohort of physicians.

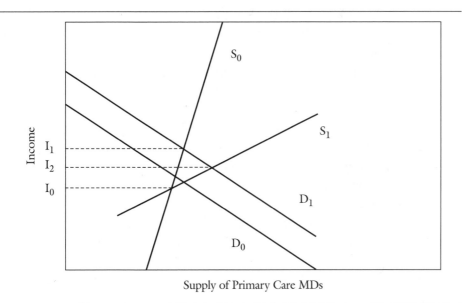

FIGURE 9.4

Short-run and Long-run Responses to Demand Shifts

The increase in the financial attractiveness of primary care was not lost on medical students, however. Increasing numbers of them entered primary care residencies after the incomes of primary care physicians began to rise (and the incomes of some subspecialists began to drop). Eventually, this will shift out the supply of primary care physicians from S_0 to S_1. As Figure 9.4 makes clear, when these additional physicians begin to practice, primary care physicians' incomes will drop (from I_1 to I_2). This appears to correspond to the recent slump in primary care physicians' incomes.

S_L represents the supply of primary care services in the long run, which is far more elastic than either of the short-run supply curves, because additional students can enter primary care specialties in response to higher incomes. Typically, the longer the time period involved, the more elastic is supply.

9.3 Who Pays for Health Insurance?

Most managers believe that because their organization writes the check to a health insurer, the organization "pays" for health insurance (and that a rise in health insurance costs would reduce profits or force the organization to raise prices). Most economists, however, believe that the workers "pay" for health insurance (and that a rise in health insurance costs would drive down wages). The logic of supply and demand analysis explains why economists make this prediction, and we will use it to explore the impact of a health insurance employer mandate on wages and employment.

The number of Americans without health insurance is growing; and because many of them are employed, a number of employer mandates have been proposed. An employer mandate would require that an employer offer at least a minimal health insurance package to all employees. Typically the employer would also be required to pay part of the cost of the insurance plan. What would the economic effects of an employer mandate be?

This turns out to be a complex question, yet analysis of demand and supply curves yields some important insights. Suppose that the government mandates that every employer offer every employee health insurance worth I. Most employers focus on total compensation per worker and, at least initially, would be unwilling to have the mandate increase total compensation. We assume, therefore, that employers who do not now offer insurance reduce salaries by I. Other sequences, including ones involving employment cuts rather than pay cuts, lead ultimately to the same conclusions.

By focusing on employers who do not offer health insurance, we will discover that the effects of the mandate depend on two factors. The first is how much health insurance is worth to these employees. The second is how responsive the supply of labor is to changes in wage rates (i.e., the elasticity of supply of labor).

If workers view health insurance that costs I as worth exactly I, there is no story to tell. Workers will perceive that the demand for labor has not shifted, only the composition of compensation. Wages will be lower, benefits will be higher, and employment will remain unchanged. Workers bear the full cost of the mandate.

To highlight what will happen in other cases, we focus on workers who view the health insurance benefit as having no worth to them personally (such as a worker with full coverage from a spouse). Figure 9.5 portrays workers who think that health insurance is worthless, so they perceive that their wage has fallen by I. From their perspective, the demand for labor has shifted from $D(W,P)$ to $D(W - I,P)$, where W is the wage, and P is the price of output in their sector. As a result, the going wage will fall from W_0 to W_1 and employment will drop from

FIGURE 9.5

Wage Effects When Workers Do Not Want Health Insurance

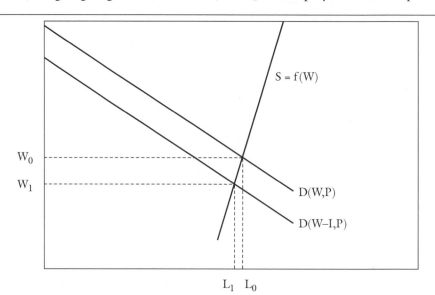

L_0 to L_1. If employment changes very little in response to the drop in wages (as Figure 9.5 suggests), equilibrium wages will drop by nearly I, employment will drop by only a little, and employers will experience little or no rise in labor costs. $W_1 + I$ is only a little more than W_0. As we will see, the elasticity of the supply of labor is one of the key issues that determines who bears the burden of a tax or regulation.

Figure 9.6 also describes the behavior of workers who think that health insurance is worthless. Here, however, workers reduce hours supplied rather substantially in response to the drop in wages. As a result, the going wage will fall from W_0 to W_1 and employment will drop from L_0 to L_1. If employment changes substantially in response to the drop in wages (as Figure 9.6 suggests), wages will drop by much less than I, employment will drop considerably, and employers will experience major increases in labor costs. This is the case in which employers "pay" for a major portion of health insurance costs: workers attach no value to health insurance and the supply of labor is very elastic.

This analysis tells us that managers need two forms of information: how much their workers value health insurance and how responsive their supply of labor is to wages. A number of studies confirm that for most workers, the supply of labor is not very responsive to changes in wages. Most people have to work. Some, however, have options that are nearly as good as their current level of participation in the paid labor force. For example, some college students can work more and take fewer classes or vice versa. Alternatively, some parents could work more, or choose to spend more time taking care of their children. These workers may respond to fairly small changes in wages. An employer whose workers might want to reduce their hours in response to a drop in cash compensation and whose workers assign little value to health insurance should anticipate that the mandate would increase labor costs noticeably. Most employers facing this situation would oppose an employer mandate, as it would reduce their profits.

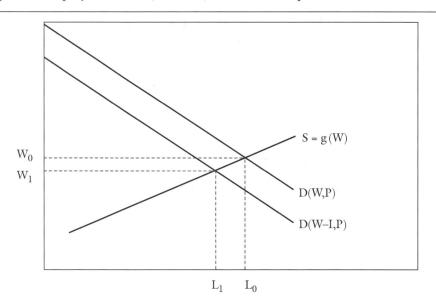

FIGURE 9.6
Wage Effects When Workers Do Not Want Health Insurance and the Supply of Labor is Elastic

As for the question, "Who pays for health insurance benefits?", the answer is dependent on how much employees want health insurance and on their elasticity of supply of labor.

9.4 Conclusion

Supply and demand analyses let managers anticipate the effects of changes in markets. Even with relatively limited data, managers can sketch the impact of a policy change on prices and volumes. Demand and supply analyses can give managers a vitally important overview of their markets and make better strategic decisions possible.

Only a few factors shift demand or supply curves. Demand curves shift right (meaning that more will be demanded at every price or that higher prices will be offered at each quantity) when incomes rise, insurance coverage expands, the prices of substitutes rise, or the prices of complements fall. Supply curves shift right (meaning that more will be supplied at every price or that lower prices will be sought at each quantity) when input prices fall, technology improves, or regulations ease.

Shifts in demand and supply curves change equilibrium prices and quantities. When a demand curve shifts to the right, equilibrium prices and quantities both rise. When a supply curve shifts to the right, equilibrium prices fall and equilibrium quantities rise. In either case, the details of the new equilibrium depend on the slope of the other curve.

References

Rizzo, J. A., and D. Blumenthal. 1994. "Physician Labor Supply: Do Income Effects Matter?" *Journal of Health Economics* 13 (4): 433–53.

Simon, C. J., D. Dranove, and W. D. White. 1998. "The Effect of Managed Care on the Incomes of Primary Care and Specialty." *Health Services Research* 33 (3, part I): 549–69.

PRICING

Key Concepts

- Pricing is important.
- **Marginal cost pricing** uses estimates of the price elasticity of demand and incremental costs to set the profit-maximizing price.
- Marginal cost pricing maximizes profits in most cases.
- The consequences of setting price incorrectly can be substantial.
- **Price discrimination**—charging different customers different prices for the same product—is common in healthcare, as it is in other industries.
- Price discrimination can substantially increase profits.
- Contracting demands the same information as pricing.

10.1 Introduction

Pricing is important. Prices that are too low or too high will drag down profits. The trick is to set prices so that your organization captures profitable business and discourages unprofitable business. To maximize profits, firms should set prices so that marginal revenue just equals marginal cost (assuming that the product line is profitable). To maximize other objectives, organizations should use profit-maximizing prices as the starting point.

Pricing represents a continuing challenge for healthcare organizations for three reasons. First, many managers do not have a clear pricing strategy. As a result, they lack the data that they need to make good decisions and may be mispricing their products or selling the wrong product lines. Second, many healthcare organizations have jumped directly from the hothouse of cost-plus or reimbursement-plus pricing to the real world of competitive bidding and negotiated contracts. Therefore, many organizations lack the skills and experience to set prices and negotiate contracts. Third, the pricing strategy that is best for the organization may not be the best for specific departments or clinics. Managers of these units may have incentives to price products too high or too low. In the absence of a clear strategy and good data, how prices will actually be set is often unclear.

10.2 The Economic Model of Pricing

The economic model of pricing, which is called **marginal cost pricing**, clearly identifies a pricing strategy that will maximize profits. This pricing strategy also identifies the information needed to set prices, simplifying the process.

The economic model of pricing is quite simple. First, find out what your incremental (or marginal) costs are. Second, estimate the price elasticity of demand facing your organization's product. (Demand for the products of your organization will usually be much more elastic than the overall demand for the product.) Third, use this information to calculate the appropriate markup, which will equal $\varepsilon/(1 + \varepsilon)$, where ε represents the price elasticity of demand for your organization's product. The pricing rule is just a restatement of the profit maximization rule, which requires equating marginal revenue and marginal cost. Marginal revenue equals $P \times (1 + \varepsilon)/\varepsilon$, so the marginal cost pricing rule emerges when you rearrange MR = MC. Multiplying this markup by your organization's incremental cost gives you the profit-maximizing price, which will equal $\varepsilon/(1 + \varepsilon) \times MC$. Therefore, if the price elasticity of demand is −2.5 and the incremental cost is $3.00, the profit-maximizing price would be $-2.5/(1 - 2.5) \times 3.00$, or $5.00.

Data on incremental costs are important for a wide range of management decisions. Pricing is just one more reason to estimate incremental costs. Estimating the right price elasticity of demand can be more of a challenge. Three strategies can provide you with this information.

1. Hire a marketing consultant. Depending on how much your organization is willing to spend, the consultant can provide you with either a rough or a fairly detailed estimate.
2. Combine information on overall price elasticities of demand with information on your market share for this product line. Dividing the overall price elasticity of demand by your market share gives an estimate of the price elasticity that your organization faces. For example, if the overall price elasticity is −0.3 and your organization commands an eighth of the market, you would estimate that your organization faces a price elasticity of demand of −0.3/0.125, or −2.4.
3. Experiment. For example, raise a product's price by 5 percent and see how much demand falls. Since the price elasticity of demand equals the percentage change in quantity divided by the percentage change in price, this calculation is straightforward.

Figure 10.1 shows that profit-maximizing markups can be quite different. An organization facing a price elasticity of demand of −2.5 and an incremental cost of $10.00 should have a markup of $6.67. In contrast, a similar organization facing a price elasticity of demand of −5.5 should set a markup of $2.22. Each of these choices maximizes profits, given the market environment that each firm faces. Clearly, organizations that face less elastic demand enjoy larger markups. Differentiated products face less elastic demand, so the payoffs to differentiating your products can be substantial.

Elasticity	Price
−1.5	$30.00
−2.5	16.67
−3.5	14.00
−4.5	12.86
−5.5	12.22
−6.5	11.82
−7.5	11.54
−8.5	11.33
−9.5	11.18

FIGURE 10.1
Profit-maximizing Prices when Incremental Costs Equal $10

10.3 Pricing and Profits

What should you do if the rate of return from a line of business is inadequate? The obvious thing to do is to raise prices. Unfortunately, like many seemingly obvious answers, this one will often be wrong. If a product line yields an inadequate return on investment, four strategies should be explored.

1. Make sure that your price is not too high or too low. Either could be the culprit if your estimate of marginal cost or the price elasticity of demand are inaccurate.
2. Reassess your estimate of incremental costs. If your estimate of incremental cost is too high, your prices will also be too high. If your estimate of incremental cost is too low, your prices will also be too low.
3. See how much your costs can be cut. Most healthcare firms should be able to reduce their costs quite substantially. To see whether your costs can be brought down, take a look at costs and business practices in firms that you think are efficient.
4. If all else fails, exit the line of business.

The consequences of setting price incorrectly can be substantial. In Figure 10.2, the profit-maximizing price should be $15.00. Setting a price much lower or much higher than $15.00 reduces profits significantly. Note, however, that being slightly high or low is not usually disastrous. Being a little off in your estimates of incremental cost or the price elasticity of demand will usually mean that your profits will be only slightly effected.

Pricing is an important component of marketing. How is the marginal cost pricing model that has been outlined above too simple? The main concern is that the marginal cost pricing model does not really consider strategic possibilities. For example, demand for an innovative product will typically be less elastic than the demand for other products. The resulting high margins, unfortunately, will

FIGURE 10.2

Profits when
Incremental and
Average Costs
Equal $10 and the
Price Elasticity of
Demand Equals
−3.0

Price	Profits
$5.00	($881,059)
7.50	(130,527)
10.00	0
12.50	28,194
15.00	32,632
17.50	30,824
20.00	27,533
22.50	24,172
25.00	21,145

attract a host of rivals. Your organization may want to forego some immediate profits to discourage entry by competitors. Alternatively, aggressive price cutting in mature markets is likely to encourage price cutting by your competitors. In markets with relatively few competitors, showing that your organization will not "rock the boat" by lowering prices may allow everyone to enjoy stable, high prices and profits. There are many options to be considered, however, and even when you do not follow the marginal cost-pricing scenario, it should be your starting point.

10.4 Price Discrimination

Price discrimination is common in healthcare, as it is in other industries. **Price discrimination** refers to charging different customers different prices for the same product. Price discrimination makes sense if different customers have different price elasticities of demand and if resale by customers is not possible. Most healthcare firms meet these criteria. They contract with an array of individuals and insurance plans. The price sensitivities of those purchasers differ widely, and services can seldom be resold. Therefore, profit-maximizing healthcare firms will want to explore opportunities for price.

Different Discounts for Different Customers

What do American Airlines, Glaxo Wellcome, Staples, Stanford University, AT&T, the Mayo Clinic, and Safeway have in common? They all price discriminate, says Scott Woolley (1998), charging different customers different amounts for the same product.

In addition, Woolley forecasts that price discrimination will increase in both frequency and complexity, as information systems allow both buyers and sellers to expand price discrimination. Right now buyers can use computers to search for price differences and demand the lowest price available. For example, Priceline.com allows customers to shop for discounted airline tickets over the Internet. Jay S. Walker, its founder, argues that the steady drop in the costs of information processing will allow a massive expansion of price discrimination. Sellers will be able to use detailed information about individual customers to offer the price-conscious ones substantial discounts while asking "big spenders" to pay list prices. Instead of just charging vacationers less than business travelers, firms may offer some individual vacationers bigger discounts than others.

Primitive versions of these tactics already exist. Victoria's Secret sends out catalogs with higher prices to customers in affluent ZIP codes. Staples goes so far as to send different catalogs with different prices to its customers. Thrifty customers track these differences and pay the lower prices, while those who do not pay more.

The information age not only makes price discrimination easier, it also makes it more important. Price discrimination makes more sense when some customers are substantially more price-sensitive than others. It may be vital when fixed costs are high relative to variable costs. Price discrimination allows firms to earn high margins on full-price sales while increasing volume via discounted sales. Both high margins and increased volume allow firms with substantial fixed costs to be profitable. And, of course, complex information systems represent a substantial new category of fixed costs.

How you price discriminate matters. The trick is to have list prices that virtually no one pays and to offer different customers different discounts. Consumers are annoyed by getting a smaller discount than their neighbor, but are infuriated by paying more than list.

If you think that price discrimination is a trick played only by major corporations, you are wrong. The sliding fee schedule in your local community clinic is another example—if it did not charge some customers more than its poorest customers could afford, the clinic would probably have to close.

Price discrimination can sharply increase profits. Suppose that half of your customers (Group A) have price elasticities of −3.00 and half (Group B) have price elasticities of −6.00. Your average and incremental cost is $10. In setting prices you could use the average price elasticity of demand (−4.50) and charge everyone $12.86. Or, you could charge Group A $12.00 and charge Group B $15.00 (which is what the marginal cost pricing model tells us to do). Figure 10.3 shows how not price discriminating leaves a substantial amount on the table.

10.4.1 Cost Shifting

Aside from managers (who are eager to learn new ways to improve profits) and consumers (who are eager to learn new ways to get discounts), why should price discrimination matter to anyone else? It is because some observers think that the different prices that they see reflect **cost shifting**, not price discrimination. According to the cost-shifting hypothesis, price reductions negotiated by PPOs

FIGURE 10.3
Profits With and
Without Price
Discrimination

Price	Quantity	Profit	Group	Price	Quantity	Profit
$12.86	9,213	$26,349	A	$15.00	5,250	$26,250
			B	$12.00	5,700	$7,800
Totals	9,213	$26,349			10,950	$34,050

or imposed by Medicaid will raise costs for everybody else. The cost-shifting hypothesis is widely believed. For example, in 1994 the *New York Times* reported that 10–30 percent of private premiums are paid to cover the costs of people who don't have health insurance (Clymer 1994).

While the cost-shifting hypothesis might be true, there are three possibilities. First, the cost-shifting hypothesis may be a rationalization for widespread discounting. No customers like getting the smallest discounts. Healthcare firms can divert attention from their profit-seeking activities by changing the subject. This is the most likely scenario, as most of the empirical evidence from the contemporary marketplace is inconsistent with the cost-shifting hypothesis (Morrisey 1994).

Second, cost shifting might be real, reflecting poor management on the part of profit-seeking organizations. If a firm raised prices to some customers because other customers negotiated a discount, it either set prices too low to begin with or was acting imprudently in raising prices.

Third, cost shifting might be real, reflecting responses of not-for-profit firms that had set prices lower than a well-managed, for-profit firm would have. Pressure on the bottom lines of contemporary healthcare organizations would suggest that even if it was practiced at one time, cost shifting is probably a thing of the past.

Pharmacy Pricing

With concern increasing about rapidly rising pharmaceutical costs, why would anyone without stock in a drug company oppose letting the nation's public hospitals take advantage of discounts that the federal government has already negotiated? Lisa Scott reports that hospitals that will not be eligible for the discounts fear that their costs will rise if public hospitals are allowed to use federal supply schedules, which could reduce their drug acquisition costs by up to 16 percent (1996). Therefore, whether federal discounts reflect price termination or cost shifting could have million-dollar consequences. If these federal discounts represent price discrimination, private sector drug costs should not change (and might even fall). If the cost-shifting argument of the Health Industry Group Purchasing Association is correct, however, bigger discounts for public hospitals could significantly increase costs for private hospitals.

Federal supply schedules list products on which the government has negotiated a price break, and there are several. The federal government buys over $2.5 billion in drugs and medical supplies each year (about 5 percent of total hospital supply purchases in the United States). In contrast, Scott's report in *Modern Healthcare* estimates that Premiere, the largest private hospital alliance, accounts for 15 to 18 percent of hospital supply spending (1996).

Will larger discounts for public hospitals mean smaller discounts for private hospitals? Probably not. The Health Industry Group Purchasing Association's prediction implies that managers of pharmaceutical firms are doing a bad job. After all, if it is profitable to raise drug prices after the public hospitals become eligible for these discounts, it should be profitable to raise drug prices now. Pharmaceutical firms should already be charging private hospitals the prices that maximize profits. Prices above the profit-maximizing level will actually reduce pharmaceutical firms' profits, and no one contends that the drug companies are not seeking to maximize profits.

An earlier analysis done on behalf of the Health Industry Group Purchasing Association predicted that drug prices would rise after Congress mandated larger Medicaid discounts. In fact, the rate of increase in drug prices slowed somewhat.

Whether we see such tactics as cost shifting or price discrimination is not just a semantic argument. Each predicts very different responses by healthcare providers when an HMO gets a big price break or when Medicare reduces its fees. Cost shifting predicts that the fees paid by other insurers will rise. Price discrimination predicts that the fees paid by other insurers will not change (and may fall). Discounts are often large. Morrisey estimated that in 1990, Medicaid paid $550 per day for hospital care, Medicare paid $615, and private insurers paid $876 (1994).

These same sorts of differences are also common in other industries with similar characteristics. Have you ever wondered why it makes sense for one passenger to have paid $340 for his flight and another passenger in the same row to have paid $99? Why does it make sense for a "twilight" screening of a movie to cost half as much as the same show two hours later? Because when the incremental cost of production is small, when buyers can be separated into groups that have very different price elasticities of demand, and when resale is not possible, price discrimination is usually profitable. Most healthcare firms fit this profile, so their managers need to know how to price discriminate. This is true for both not-for-profit and for-profit organizations alike. With no margin, there is no mission. Price discrimination helps increase margins.

10.5 Multi-Part Pricing

Thus far we have focused on simple pricing models, when in fact, there are a wide range that may be applicable. One is the **multi-part pricing** model, in which model customers pay a fee to be eligible to use a service and separate fees to use services. An obvious example would be a managed care plan. The trade-off is that a low entry fee (premium) yields more customers. High co-pays reduce costs (hence either increase profit margins or reduce premiums), but at some point high co-pays will drive away customers. The right combination is always a balancing act. A related pricing strategy is called **tying**. Tying links the prices of multiple products. Again, the goal is to balance multiple prices so as to maximize profits.

10.6 Pricing and Managed Care

Are these issues relevant in markets dominated by managed care? Yes. One needs the same information to set a price or evaluate a contract. It almost never makes sense to accept a contract in which marginal revenue is less than incremental cost. Contracts that increase an organization's losses, which is what happens when marginal revenue is less than incremental costs, make sense only when these losses are really marketing expenses. Even in these cases there are usually less costly marketing strategies. Similarly, it almost never makes sense to give a large discount to a buyer who is price insensitive. For example, a managed care plan that needs your organization to offer a competitive network is not in a good bargaining position and should not get the best discount.

What should my firm bid for this contract?

Shahram Heshmat points out that the answer to this question is what an increasing number of healthcare managers need to know (1996). The flip side of the pricing problem, it is an even tougher dilemma. Economic models of pricing tell us that managers need to know what their incremental costs are, what markup over incremental costs they should expect, and what their rivals will bid. Each of these will be uncertain to some degree.

Data on costs should be within the grasp of every firm, but many healthcare organizations have only sketchy data. This is especially true for incremental costs, which many are not prepared to track. Without good data on incremental costs, managers may be tempted to base their bids on average costs. This usually forfeits some profitable business opportunities.

The right markup is always a strategic decision, but managers must avoid the temptation to turn the job into a "loss leader." In the heat of the battle, there is a temptation to low-ball the markup to increase your chances of winning the bid. Winning contracts that lose money seldom makes companies profitable or gets managers promoted

Who will bid is the real wild card. Most of the time, healthcare providers know who their rivals will be and how much they want the contract. Many government contracts require that potential bidders identify themselves in advance, and a list of potential bidders is usually available to all those on the list. For major contracts, managers will also call their sources to find out how serious some of their potential rivals are (and spread some misinformation about their own interest).

Before submitting your best-and-final bid, remember that the winning bidder in an auction often winds up regretting it. After all, in a competitive environment, firms that have underestimated their costs are the most likely to submit the low bid.

10.7 Conclusion

Pricing is important, but many healthcare firms are flying blind, lacking a clear model of pricing. Managers do not really know what their incremental costs are and they do not know what sort of price elasticity of demand their organization faces. As a result, they do not know what price to charge, reducing profits in two ways: the organization may have set its prices too high or too low, or the organization may be participating in the wrong markets. It may be accepting contracts that it should refuse or it may be refusing contracts that it should accept.

The economic model of pricing tells managers what they should do. Its implications, moreover, apply to both pricing and contracting, making it an important part of every healthcare manager's skill set. Actually applying this model will not always be easy, but not knowing what to do is even more difficult.

Price discrimination is everywhere in healthcare, and many organizations rely on it to remain profitable. To do so, price discriminating requires a little more information than setting a single price, so the above comments apply with greater force. In addition, many healthcare managers appear to be mesmerized by tales of cost shifting. Cost shifting represents a useful public relations ploy, because it reduces the dissatisfaction of those paying list price. Remember, however, that cost shifting may or may not be a realistic practice, and can steer managers in the wrong direction.

References

Clymer, A. 1994. "In the Arithmetic of Health Care, it Pays to Aim for 100%." *New York Times* July 24, E16.

Heshmat, S. 1996. "A Decision Model for Competitive Bidding: Price Negotiations for the Health Care Industry." *Journal of Health Care Finance* 22 (4): 81–87.

Morrisey, M. 1994. *Cost Shifting in Health Care: Separating Evidence from Rhetoric* Washington, D.C.: AEI Press.

Scott, L. 1996. "Government Buying Play Provokes Private Sector." *Modern Healthcare* November 11, 56.

Woolley, S. 1998. "I Got it Cheaper than You." *Forbes* 162 (10): 82–84.

ASYMMETRIC INFORMATION AND INCENTIVES

Key Concepts

- **Asymmetric information** is present when one party to a transaction has better information about it than another.
- Asymmetric information makes it possible for the better-informed party to act opportunistically.
- Aligning incentives helps reduce the problems associated with asymmetric information.
- Concerns about risk, complexity, measurement problems, strategic responses, and team production limit incentive-based payments.
- Only a few forms of incentive-based contracts are common in healthcare.

11.1 Asymmetric Information

Asymmetric information confronts healthcare managers in most of their professional roles. Consider several examples:

- Vendors typically know more about the strengths and weaknesses of their products than do purchasers.
- Employees typically know more about their health problems than do human resource or health plan managers.
- Subordinates typically know more about the effort that they have put into their assignments than do their superiors.
- Providers typically know more about the treatment options than do their patients.

In all of these examples, one party, commonly called an **agent**, has better information than another party, commonly called a **principal**. Unless the principal is careful, the agent may take advantage of this information asymmetry. Doing so is called **opportunism**.

Asymmetric information can result in two types of problems. One is that mutually beneficial transactions may not take place if concern about it is too great. The other is that resources may be wasted because of opportunism on the part of agents or costly precautions on the part of principals. For example, consumers may not use mental health services because their health plan limits coverage to prevent abuse. Alternatively, costs may be driven up because providers bill for services of questionable value or because the plan requires prior authorization for all services.

Asymmetric information affects managers directly in other ways. Senior management may be unwilling to give unit managers enough authority to run their units well, fearing that managers may boost their profits by reducing service to other units. Senior management may also feel the need to monitor the performance of the units via internal audits and inspections. Both of these increase costs without directly adding to the output of the organization. The implications of asymmetric information are far reaching.

Three conditions must be present for asymmetric information to be a concern:

1. The interests of the parties must diverge in some meaningful way.
2. There must be some important reason for the parties to strike a deal.
3. There must be difficulties in determining whether the explicit or implicit terms of the deal have been followed.

These circumstances are far from rare. Unfortunately, they represent an invitation to act opportunistically.

11.2 Opportunism

Opportunism can take many forms, such as deliberately billing a health plan for services that were not actually rendered (known as fraud). But the forms of opportunism that managers must deal with are not usually so stark: employees surfing the Internet rather than making collection calls; using the supplies budget to refurbish an office; scheduling a physical therapy visit of questionable value to meet volume targets; or referring a patient to a specialist for a problem that the primary care physician could easily handle.

Experience forces us to assume that some individuals are opportunistic some of the time. As a first step, we try to avoid dealing with those who are the most opportunistic. We then try to set up systems to restrain opportunistic behavior. These systems will be imperfect, however, because of our inability to anticipate what may happen and how individuals may react.

Remedies for asymmetric information focus on aligning the interests of the parties or on monitoring the behavior of the agent. Changes in incentives are usually at least a part of the preferred strategy, because monitoring agents is typically expensive and nonproductive. For example, healthcare plans commonly have utilization review procedures that are designed to control use of services. However, because most utilization review does not change the recommended therapy, despite its cost and annoyance, health plans would love to be in a position to eliminate the entire utilization review process. A plan that could do so would rapidly gain market share, as it could increase consumer and provider satisfaction and reduce premiums. In addition to being costly, monitoring may be quite difficult. For example, a product that a vendor honestly recommended may fail or may not meet your unique needs. Or it may work, but have unneeded capabilities and cost far more than a more suitable product would. Monitoring is likely to be only a part of the response to asymmetric information.

The challenges posed by asymmetric information are not unique to health-care, although their extent does pose special problems for managers. Three features make asymmetric information especially troublesome in the healthcare sector:

1. In paying the bills of healthcare providers, insurance creates a principal-agent relationship that is not found in most fields.
2. Insurance also sharply reduces the patient's incentive to monitor the performance of healthcare providers, as it limits the patient's financial exposure to opportunism.
3. Asymmetric information lies at the heart of most provider-patient relationships. Patients typically seek out providers because they want information, so the threat of opportunism is always there.

These three problems, when added to the garden-variety forms of oppor-tunism that can be found in most systems, demand that healthcare managers directly confront the challenges posed by asymmetric information.

Of course, opportunism is such an obvious risk that institutions appear to have developed ways to limit it (Arrow 1963). One of the most obvious is the preference for dealing with those who have proven themselves. For example, primary care physicians tend to refer patients to physicians who have served them and their patients well in the past. Knowing this, even a specialist who might be tempted to provide unnecessary services to a patient will be reluctant to do so. These sorts of ongoing relationships—between buyer and seller, between patient and provider, or between supervisor and subordinate—tend to deter observable opportunism. Much of the regulation of the healthcare sector can also be seen as an attempt to deter opportunism. The problem is that both of these mechanisms require that opportunism be detectable. In many cases it is not.

11.2.1 Signaling

When differences in quality or other attributes of care are hard to observe, agents may seek to send signals that reassure principals. These signals should tell prospective clients about the agent, should be hard to counterfeit, and should be relatively inexpensive. Brand names are classic signals. It costs relatively little to put a Pfizer label on a new drug, but consumers who are not well informed can be reassured that the drug will meet stringent quality standards because substandard quality will hurt Pfizer's worldwide sales. The challenge is to pre-vent others from counterfeiting the labels. One of the puzzles of the healthcare market is why branding, especially branding of healthcare services, is not more common.

Quality certification is another strategy for dealing with asymmetric in-formation. Hospitals that are accredited by the Joint Commission on the Ac-creditation of Healthcare Organizations send a clear signal of quality that is very difficult to counterfeit. Unfortunately, the process is so expensive that many smaller hospitals do not seek accreditation.

Other signals may be of use as well, but are likely to be less credible. For example, high prices and high levels of advertising also serve as quality signals, as the sales losses that result from high prices are especially damaging for low-cost, low-quality products (Bagwell and Riordan 1991). In markets with standardized products, poorly informed agents can buy information (e.g., by subscribing to *Consumer Reports*) or copy well-informed agents. The more individualized the product, however, the less this strategy works, so its value is unclear in much of healthcare. Therefore, while we can identify healthcare cases in which signaling reduces the problems associated with differential information, it is far from a comprehensive solution. Improving information is likely to leave significant residual gaps.

11.3 Incentive Problems

Incentive problems are pervasive, so managing in the face of important information asymmetries requires careful attention to incentives. Consider the case of a firm that wants its managers to promote a safe working environment (presumably because it is more profitable than an unsafe one). A salaried manager has only a limited incentive to ensure that the work environment is safe. Unsafe work practices often boost production, and promoting safety may well divert the manager from marketing or cost-reduction efforts that could boost the unit's profits. Promotions and salary increases usually await those who increase profits, not those who run the safest unit. Poor safety hurts the organization's profits (because workers' compensation premiums rise), but may not hurt the unit's profits, because the workers' compensation plan covers the entire organization.

Analysis of an Incentive Scheme

An analysis of an incentive scheme demonstrates the effects of putting managers at risk for outcomes that they imperfectly control (Puelz and Snow 1997). A restaurant chain switched from a fixed salary for managers to a contract that paid a fixed wage plus a share of the restaurant's profits, with a penalty for workers' compensation claims. The penalty was $500 per claim for claims below $500 and $1,700 for all higher claims. Such an incentive system rewards managers who improve the safety of their workplace. It also gives managers incentives not to report accidents, even though the contract also made them liable for any fines assessed by the Occupational Safety and Health Administration for false reports.

Not surprisingly, the incentive contract reduced reported claims, which dropped by 77 percent, while the dollar value of claims per restaurant dropped by 69 percent. Because inexpensive claims (like burns or lacerations) and expensive claims (like sprains and hernias) both dropped, the authors infer managers actually were able to reduce the number of accidents, although the evidence is not conclusive. It appears that fewer accidents were reported, as the average cost per claim rose by nearly 50 percent.

This example illustrates both the power and limits of using incentives to influence the behavior of agents. Incentives often elicit quite significant changes in observed behavior, but what the agent actually does may not correspond perfectly to the principal's intentions.

11.4 Incentive Design for Providers

To a large extent the growth of managed care represents a recognition that the insurance system of the United States creates multiple incentives for inefficiency. Providers were faced with strong incentives to provide care as long as the benefits exceeded the cost to their patients, and costly care was often free for insured patients. Neither party had a compelling reason for taking the true cost of care into account. We have already discussed redesign of consumer payments, so this chapter will focus on how providers are paid.

Let us begin with an examination of the incentives implicit in the four most common methods for paying providers: fee-for-service payments, salaries, capitation, and case rates. We will see that each of these methods has some advantages and disadvantages.

Figure 11.1 contrasts the incentives created by different pure payment systems. Note that fee-for-service and salary compensation systems incorporate incentives that are polar opposites. Capitation and case-rate systems have quite similar incentive structures that fall between the two polar cases. Fee-for-service, case rate, and capitation payment systems immediately reward providers who have large numbers of clients. More clients mean higher revenues with all of these systems. In contrast, unless other incentive systems are in place (such as review by superiors or the possibility for promotions) salary and budget payment systems do not reward providers who add clients. The only form of payment that rewards

	Fee-for-service	Case rates	Capitation	Salary or budget
Number of clients	+	+	+	−
Services per client	+	−	−	−
Client acuity*	+	−	−	−
Unbillable services**	−	+	+	+

FIGURE 11.1 Financial Incentives of Alternative Compensation Systems

A + indicates that the compensation scheme rewards producing more of an output or using more of an input. A − indicates that the compensation scheme rewards producing less of an output or using less of an input.
* In this context client acuity refers to the amount of services that a client is likely to need. Higher acuity means a client is likely to need more services.
** Unbillable services include both services for which the provider cannot bill because of the provisions of the insurance plan and services provided by others.

those who provide a large volume of services per client is fee-for-service payment. In case-rate and capitation systems the disincentive for high levels of service per client is tempered by the rewards of attracting additional clients. Clients expect service, so providers need to be careful in reducing services per client. Again, salary or budget systems do not reward high levels of service per client.

All of the payment systems except fee-for-service contain an incentive to avoid clients with complicated, expensive problems (or at least to prefer clients with simple, inexpensive problems). Expensive clients, when combined with fixed payments per case or per period, are financially unrewarding for providers. In like fashion, all of the payment systems except fee-for-service contain an incentive to use external services (such as church-sponsored organizations or services provided by friends) as long as they are cost effective from the perspective of providers. There is likely to be an incentive to refer too much, especially if the provider does not bear the full costs of the services of community organizations or other providers. In contrast, under fee-for-service payment only billable services can be profitable. Fee-for-service creates an incentive not to use external resources (or at least not to use the organization's resources to improve clients' access to them). Fee-for-service typically rewards providers who refer too little, from society's perspective.

None of these payment systems solve the asymmetric information problem. Providers will still usually know more about the treatment options that are appropriate for individual patients than either patients or insurers. Fee-for-service providers inclined to opportunism will still be able to recommend additional billable services; case-rate providers inclined to opportunism will still be able to avoid unprofitable cases; capitated providers inclined to opportunism will still be able to recommend very limited treatment plans; and salaried providers inclined to opportunism will still be able to limit how much they do.

This discussion should not be construed as an assertion that only financial incentives matter. Such an assertion would be inconsistent with basic economic theory, which postulates that principals and agents balance alternative objectives. Only some of these goals will be financial in nature. Yet economics anticipates an aggregate response to financial incentives nonetheless. For example, because of their commitment to the health of their patients or because it is an effective marketing tool, some physicians may offer extensive patient education programs, even if the fee-for-service payment system does not treat this as a billable service. Economics does predict that physicians will offer more of such services if the fee-for-service payment system offers compensation for them or if they are profitable under case-rate or capitation arrangements.

Suppose that a physician schedules four patients per hour for 30 hours per week (Kralewski et al. 1998), as in Figure 11.2. Under Plan A he realizes a $20 compensation per patient and has a total income of $115,200. (Basing compensation on visits is designed to simplify our discussion, not define an attractive fee-for-service compensation plan. More sensible fee-for-service systems base compensation on billings, relative value units, and the like.) Plan B incorporates a base salary of $80,000 plus $20 per patient for visits in excess of 4,000. At

Plan	Base salary	Marginal compensation	Volume payments	Total income
A	$0	$20	$115,200	$115,200
B	80,000	20	35,200	115,200
C	100,000	20	35,200	135,200
D	57,600	10	57,600	115,200

FIGURE 11.2
An Illustrative
Model of Incentives

the margin, plans A and B have the same incentives, even though B combines salary and volume-based payments. Each pays $20 for seeing one more patient and affords the physician the same total income. This is important because mixed compensation systems can give agents similar incentives with less risk than pure compensation systems.

The incentives of Plan C, which offers a $100,000 base salary plus $20 per patient for visits in excess of 4,000, are subtly different from the incentives in Plans A and B. Although paying $20 per visit at the margin, the physician's income will be higher under C than if he saw the same number of patients under Plans A or B. This "income effect" may reduce his willingness to add an additional patient at the end of the day or double book in order to squeeze in an acutely ill patient. Income effects mean that the effects of incentive systems need not be straightforward, although they usually are (Rizzo and Blumenthal 1994).

Plan D has quite different incentives. It offers a base salary of $57,600 plus $10 for each patient visit. Even though the physician's income will be the same if he sees 5,760 patients per year under Plans A, B, and D, he is likely to see fewer patients under Plan D because the marginal reward is so much smaller.

11.4.1 Managed Care and Incentives

Given the importance of how providers are paid, how has the growth of managed care changed compensation systems? Rather less than expected, actually. Even in areas in which managed care is pervasive most physicians continue to be paid based on their personal productivity (typically measured by billings, visits, or net revenue), just as they were before the advent of managed care (Kralewski et al 1998). In addition, even though hospital outpatient services represent one of the fastest growing components of medical spending, many health plans continue to pay hospital outpatient departments on the basis of discounted charges (Lake 1998). Only a few plans have implemented fee schedules, and fewer still have moved to case rates. Case rates (in the form of DRGs) are quite common forms of hospital payment, but few hospitals are paid via capitation. Many private insurance plans pay hospitals per day of care provided. In addition, how organizations get paid does not determine how individual providers are paid. It is quite common for a provider who is a part of a capitated organization to be paid on a fee-for-service basis. The example below illustrates how large the effects of incentives can be and how important it is to understand the incentives that decision makers actually face.

How much do physician incentives affect use of expensive services?

The answer is substantially, according to a recent study of alternative managed care plans (Josephson and Karcz 1997). One of the most interesting features of this study is its clear delineation of how much incentives differed for two cohorts of HMO physicians. One cohort of primary care physicians consisted of the partners in a capitated, multispecialty group practice that served 22,136 beneficiaries of a large New England HMO. Aside from stop-loss insurance, the physician owners of the practice were fully at risk for all use of care by these beneficiaries. Unspent capitation funds were distributed to the physicians at the end of the year, so the incentive to keep costs down was significant. The other cohort consisted of solo practice physicians who were members of three IPA HMOs. These physicians were paid on a fee-for-service basis that included a withhold of 10–20 percent. At the end of the year the proceeds of the withhold pool were split equally among the physicians, the hospital, and the HMO. These physicians faced limited risk. They could lose only their shares of the withhold pool. They also had rather limited motivation to keep costs down. Fee-for-service payments provided significant incentives to keep volumes (hence costs) up, and the split of the withhold pool weakened their incentives to limit use of costly services.

The patients of the capitated physicians used far fewer emergency department services. They averaged only 70 visits per thousand members per year. In contrast, the patients of the IPA physicians averaged more than five times as many visits, at 363 per thousand members per year. One reason for this differential was that physicians in the capitated practice operated an after-hours urgent care center to accommodate their patients. Their patients made more than 4,000 visits to the urgent care center. In addition, the physicians in the capitated practice made a concerted effort to serve walk-in patients during office hours to ensure that they did not get diverted to the emergency department. In contrast, the IPA physicians, who bore little of the high cost of emergency department care, often referred patients to the emergency department for care of unexpected minor illnesses.

Some of this difference might be due to different incentives for patients, which the study did not consider. It is quite possible that the IPA HMOs incorporated weaker incentives for patients to avoid using the emergency department. Although likely to have an impact, differences in patients' incentives cannot explain why the prepaid group practice provided comprehensive urgent care services and the IPA practices did not. The decision to provide urgent care services was made by the physicians. Capitation aligned the incentives of the physicians and the health plan, as both of them benefited by reducing use of high-cost emergency department services.

This is likely to be a case in which saving money also improves the quality of care. In addition to being expensive, care in the emergency department tends to be poorly integrated with other outpatient care. The emergency department physicians may lack timely access to patients' records, and communication with patients' primary care physicians tends to be problematic. Therefore, aligning incentives properly can be a win-win proposition for both the physicians and the patients.

11.5 Limits on Incentive-Based Payments

A number of factors limit how complete incentive-based payments can be. Concerns about risk, complexity, and team production make agents reluctant to enter into incentive-based compensation arrangements. Concerns about opportunism make principals reluctant, as a high-powered incentive system may leave them worse off if agents respond in unanticipated ways.

11.5.1 Risk

It is quite common to refer to capitation, utilization withholds, and case rate systems as risk sharing systems. This is somewhat misleading. The real goal of these systems is incentive alignment; that risks must be shared is a side effect. For example, capitation seeks to give physicians incentives to use resources wisely. Therefore, capitation succeeds if physicians avoid tests that cannot change their therapeutic plans, or if they avoid hospitalizations when there are better community treatment options. Full-risk capitation gives physicians incentives to take these types of steps.

Unfortunately, the financial risks associated with pure capitation can be quite substantial. One patient with a very rare, very expensive illness can bankrupt a solo practice; an unexpected jump in pharmaceutical prices can bankrupt a small provider-owned HMO. Because of these risks, capitation's growth has been slowed, and many organizations have sought to avoid full-risk capitation. A study of medium-sized clinics in an area with high managed care penetration found that only about 15 percent of their revenue came from full-risk capitation, about the same percentage coming from billed charges (Kralewski 1998). Indeed, even hospitals, which are better able to accept the risk contained in capitation contracts, appear to be sufficiently concerned about risk to have begun moving away from their limited involvement with capitation (Rauber 1999).

11.5.2 Complexity

Payment systems also have to be simple and comprehensible, which limits what incentive-based payment systems can try to do. If you seek to have the payment system reward physicians for keeping customer satisfaction high, MMR vaccination rates high, out-of-formulary drug use low, hospitalization rates low, hospital lengths of stay short, after-hours response times prompt, record updates prompt, and asthma follow-up appointments timely, the system is likely to be unwieldy.

Moreover, the reward associated with each component of the system is likely to be small. Providers and employees are more apt to respond to simple, comprehensible systems than to complex, confusing ones.

Adding to the complexity issue is opportunism, which limits the effects of incentive systems. An agent with better information than a principal can act in ways that harm the principal. In many cases it is quite difficult to know whether or not an agent has lived up to contract requirements. In other cases the agent may act in ways that the principal did not anticipate. For example, one response to the price reductions introduced by PPOs appears to have been an "unbundling" of services. Physicians and other providers began to bill separately for services once included in the standard office visit. Managers must anticipate opportunistic responses to incentive systems. Some will demand redesign; some will have to be tolerated to prevent the systems from becoming excessively complex.

An Example of a Complex Managed Care Plan

Managed care plans often combine payment methods. Simple strategies, such as capitation without risk adjustment or fee-for-service payments based on discounted charges, create risks that providers are reluctant to assume and incentives that insurers are reluctant to put in place. For example, the high costs of treating several patients with AIDS might well make a provider reluctant to accept capitation for populations with significant numbers of AIDS patients. An overview of the Maryland Medicaid risk-adjusted capitation system shows just how complex managed care plans can become (Weiner, et al. 1998).

The Maryland system assigns every beneficiary for whom it has claims information to one of 20 capitation categories. There are 17 diagnosis-based capitation categories with payments ranging from about $45 per month to roughly $1,100 per month. The program assigns new enrollees (for whom it does not have diagnostic data) to capitation groups based on location, age, and sex. For newborns, a special population of new enrollees, the program has a separate delivery case rate and a separate capitation rate for children under age one. In addition, the program pays a special capitation rate for beneficiaries with AIDS. (The program pays for protease inhibiting drugs and viral load testing on a fee-for-service basis.)

Despite the extensive amount of risk adjustment built into the Maryland program, the program incorporates three mechanisms for limiting the risks borne by healthcare organizations. First, the program has a hospital stop-loss provision. Healthcare organizations are responsible for only 10 percent of annual hospital costs in excess of $61,000 per beneficiary. Second, the program provides case-managed fee-for-service coverage for the roughly one percent of beneficiaries with "rare and expensive" conditions (such as spina bifida and cystic fibrosis). Third, the program also carves out a behavioral health fee-for-service program. (Persons with psychiatric diagnoses are also assigned fairly high capitation rates for general medical services.) These three provisions address the natural reluctance of healthcare organizations to assume these uncommon, but potentially devastating, financial risks.

While capitation sounds simple, setting up a capitation payment system is much more complicated than setting up a discounted charges payment system.

11.5.3 Team Production

Team production also limits the use of incentives. Production of healthcare products usually involves a number of people, and the shortcomings of one person can undermine the efforts of the entire team. For example, rudeness by one disaffected team member can negate the efforts of others to provide exemplary customer service. This interdependency can also weaken the effects of individual incentives. A worker who tries hard to do a good job or a physician who is conscientious about reducing length of stay is likely to get the message that this is not appreciated if the shortcomings of others deny them bonuses. Building and maintaining effective teams are important tasks for managers. Unless carefully structured, financial incentives tend to reward individualistic behavior, which usually weakens teams. While team financial incentives (e.g., bonuses for every member of the team when the team reaches its goals) do not reward individualism, they still tend to be relatively weak

11.6 Incentive Design for Managers

Incentives for managers can be financial or non-financial. It is important that these two incentive systems operate in tandem. Otherwise, the incentive systems may worsen the problems created by asymmetric information.

Incentive pay for managers represents a partial response to the asymmetric information problem. It usually takes the form of bonus payments, profit sharing, or stock options. In most cases these represent a fairly modest part of total compensation and they are only loosely tied to the performance of individuals. Four concepts appear to underlie this pattern (Baker et al. 1988).

1. Financial incentives can strongly motivate people to do what is rewarded. (This is the same problem that fee-for-service compensation presents us with.) Yet organizations seldom want managers to focus only on the duties that will increase their pay.
2. Managers' goals are not always clearly defined. They must respond creatively not only to any problems that arise, but position the organization to respond to problems that have not yet presented themselves as well. Writing a contract that bases performance on these types of unpredictable situations, however, is difficult.

3. The performance of most managers is hard to measure. Indeed, it is precisely when an individual's productivity becomes hard to measure that a shift away from compensation based on individual productivity makes sense. The number of patients seen is a good measure of the output of a dental hygienist; it is a poor measure of the output of the medical director of a clinic.
4. What is measurable and what is desired rarely coincide. Compensation based on measurable outputs is likely to increase opportunism, as managers react to what gets paid for rather than what is sought.

Generally, then, incentive pay for those with significant management roles needs to reflect the success of the overall organization. On balance, it appears that the dilution of incentives that results from using profit sharing or gain sharing is a reasonable price to pay for promoting team-oriented behavior. Gain sharing is like profit sharing, but can base bonuses on a broader array of outcomes. Members of a group can earn bonuses for hitting production, customer satisfaction, profit, quality, or cost targets. Group incentives may even be more effective than individual incentives in certain cases. The harder it is to identify individual contributions, the easier it is for members of the group to monitor each other, the more important it is that the group's incentives be aligned with the larger organization's, and the easier it is for the group to alter how it does its work, the more effective group incentives are likely to be.

Gain Sharing

Hospitals eager to cut costs and improve quality are exploring gain sharing as a strategy to do so (Jaklevic 1999). **Gain sharing** is a general strategy for offering rewards to those who contribute to the success of an organization. Profit sharing or stock options could be considered forms of gain sharing, but more typically gain sharing arrangements consist of bonuses paid to individuals in units that hit specified goals, such as reducing operating costs or improving patient outcomes. Used in manufacturing for years, gain sharing is a new idea in healthcare. Its major attraction is its versatility. It can be used for employees, managers, staff physicians, or independent physicians, and it can be based on a wide range of indicators.

The structure of the bonus payments can also vary (Dickenson et al 1999). For example, a gain sharing arrangement intended to spur development and adoption of an improved clinical protocol could pay bonuses to the members of the team (including the physicians); split a bonus pool between the hospital and the physicians; or pay a bonus to a clinical department, an especially attractive option in an academic medical center. At Stanford University Medical Center, for example, a quality improvement initiative set aside 10 percent of professional revenues from capitation (Hopkins 1999).

Clinical departments that succeeded in completing a clinical quality improvement project and staying within budget were eligible for these funds and additional bonuses. Not surprisingly, there was a sharp upsurge in clinical quality improvement activities, with the departments with the most to gain (or lose) taking the lead. The key is that gain sharing can work to reinforce desired patterns of behavior, even in cases where profit sharing or capitation are infeasible.

Incentive pay is only a part of an effective incentive system. Nothing in economic theory implies that individuals will not respond to opportunities to do challenging work, public celebrations of their accomplishments, or a positive review by a trusted mentor. An effective manager will consider these tools as well. Successful organizations require cooperation in management and production, so a non-financial system that rewards cooperation represents a sensible option for aligning incentives. Promotions typically combine financial and non-financial rewards. Not surprisingly, they represent an important part of the reward system in many organizations.

11.7 Conclusion

Restructuring incentives is an imperfect response to the problem of asymmetric information. The rewards of incentive systems are usually based on results, not what agents actually do, and it is clear that agents can respond opportunistically to virtually any incentive system. The challenge is to align the incentives of all the individuals in a system with the interests of its stakeholders. This is not easy. There is no magic formula, as good incentive systems must balance competing objectives. In addition, managers must anticipate that incentives may have multiple effects, that designing incentive systems will be costly, and that keeping incentive systems up to date will also be expensive.

References

Arrow, K. J. 1963. "Uncertainty and the Welfare Economics of Medical Care." *American Economic Review* 53 (5): 941–73.

Bagwell, K. and M. H. Riordan. 1991" High and Declining Prices Signal Product Quality." *American Economic Review* 81 (1): 224–39.

Baker, G. P., M. C. Jensen, K. J. Murphy. 1988. "Compensation and Incentives: Practice vs. Theory." *Journal of Finance* 43 (3): 593–616.

Dickenson, R. A., et al. 1999. "Rethinking Specialist Integration Strategy." *Healthcare Financial Management* 53 (1): 42–48.

Hopkins, J. R. 1999. "Financial Incentives for Ambulatory Care Performance Improvement." *Joint Commission Journal on Quality Improvement* 25 (5): 223–38.

Jaklevic, M. C. 1999. "Hospitals, Docs Benefit from Gainsharing." *Modern Healthcare* 29 (7): 34.

Josephson, G., and A. Karcz. 1997. "The Impact of Physician Economic Incentives on Admission Rates." *American Journal of Managed Care* 3 (1): 49–56.

Kralewski, J. E., E. C. Rich, T. Bernhardt, B. Dowd, R. Feldman, and C. Johnson. 1998. "The Organizational Structure of Medical Group Practices in a Managed Care Environment." *Health Care Management Review* 23 (2): 76–96.

Lake, T. 1998. "Current Trends in Health Plan Payment Methods for the Facility Costs of Outpatient Care." *Journal of Health Care Finance* 25 (2): 1–8.

Puelz, R. and A. Snow. 1997. "Optimal Incentive Contracting with *Ex Ante* and *Ex Post* Moral Hazards: Theory and Evidence." *Journal of Risk and Uncertainty* 14, 169–88.

Rauber, C. 1999. "De-capitating Managed Care Contracts." *Modern Healthcare* 29 (36): 52–56.

Rizzo, J. A. and D. Blumenthal. 1994. "Physician Labor Supply: Do Income Effects Matter?" *Journal of Health Economics* 13 (4): 433–53.

Weiner, J. P., A. M. Tucker, A. M. Collins, H. Fakhraei, R. Lieberman, C. Abrams, G. R. Trapnell, and J. G. Folkemer. 1998. "The Development of a Risk-Adjusted Capitation Payment System: The Maryland Medicaid Model." *Journal of Ambulatory Care Management* 21 (4): 29–52.

ECONOMIC ANALYSIS OF CLINICAL AND MANAGERIAL INTERVENTIONS

Key Concepts

- Analyses of interventions are designed to support decisions, not make them.
- Comparing the most plausible alternatives is vital. Well-done analyses will not be enlightening if we consider the wrong choices.
- Four types of analysis are common: cost minimization analysis (CMA), cost-effectiveness analysis (CEA), cost utility analysis (CUA) and cost benefit analysis (CBA).
- The simplest and most productive type of analysis is CMA.
- CBA and CUA are potentially more powerful, but pose many questions.
- **Modeling costs** entails identifying the perspective involved, the resources used, and the opportunity costs of those resources.
- Focus on the direct costs of interventions.
- Modeling benefits is the most difficult part of economic evaluation of clinical interventions.

12.1 Introduction

Until recently, economic analyses of clinical interventions were uncommon. Healthcare decision makers had little or no incentive to assess whether procedures were worth their costs, or even whether those procedures could be done more efficiently. To begin with, a fee-for-service payment system "tells" decision makers what procedures are "worth." When working in organizations that face a fee-for-service payment system, practical managers will not worry about genuinely balancing value and cost. If the fee-for-service payment system is based on the costs of individual hospitals or allows balance billing, even financial officers will find little value in detailed analyses of costs and revenues, let alone explorations of the true value of clinical services. Until recently, interest in economic analyses of clinical interventions has been much higher in countries other than the United States.

The emergence of global payment systems and the growth of capitation have dramatically increased the relevance of economic analyses of clinical interventions, now that money is at stake. In a global payment system, getting the same outcome at less cost directly increases profits. In a capitated system, the options are even greater. Getting the same outcome more cheaply still increases profits, but strategies such as increasing prevention, self care, or adherence to clinically effective protocols also can have a significant payoff. In short, the value of analyzing clinical interventions has risen sharply.

Analyses of clinical interventions ask apparently simple questions such as, "Are the benefits of this intervention greater than its costs?" and "Is this intervention better than the alternatives?" Such questions are often not easy to answer, because assessing the benefits of clinical interventions is difficult. While the second question may sound much like the first, it is easier to answer because it does not require that we explicitly assign a value to the benefits of an intervention.

These questions need to be asked because resources are scarce. Even in a wealthy society such as ours, resources are not unlimited. When an individual chooses to purchase a drug or be screened for a condition, he or she cannot use those resources for other purposes. The same is true for society. If the benefits of an EKG are smaller than the benefits of another use of that money, resources should be reallocated to those other uses. Ideally we would like to use resources to realize the maximum benefit possible. More practically, we seek to avoid pure waste and interventions that clearly have benefits that are smaller than their costs.

It is important to recognize that analyses of clinical interventions are designed to support decision making, not make decisions. By providing a framework for synthesizing and understanding information, economic analyses are designed to help decision makers avoid genuinely bad decisions.

Four types of analysis are common. Cost minimization analysis (CMA), cost-effectiveness analysis (CEA), cost utility analysis (CUA), and cost benefit analysis (CBA) are all designed to compare the costs and benefits of alternative interventions. All four techniques use the same methods to measure costs, but they use different strategies for assessing benefits.

For managers, CMA will be the most useful. Although more limited in scope than the others, it is simpler to apply. CMA answers our second question, "Is this intervention better than the alternatives?" Unfortunately, it cannot answer this question in every case. If the better alternative also costs more or if the least expensive alternative does not work as well, CMA is not helpful.

CEA extends CMA somewhat. When the better strategy costs more, CEA answers the question, "What is the cost per unit of this gain?" This simple piece of information is likely to be of genuine value to managers, as it will validate some strategies (because the cost per unit is very small) and negate others (because the cost per unit is very large). CEA does not, however, directly compare the costs and benefits of a strategy as CUA and CBA do, so it is still a more limited tool.

12.2 Cost Analysis

Before examining these four types of analysis in more detail, we will briefly review the basics of cost analysis. Measuring costs entails three tasks: identifying the perspective involved, identifying the resources used, and identifying the opportunity costs of those resources. Costs are often poorly understood (and poorly measured), even though the issues are seldom very complex.

12.2.1 Identifying Cost Perspective

Identifying a cost perspective is an essential first step. Confusion about costs usually arises because the analyst has not been clear about his or her perspective. Decision makers usually respond to the costs that they see, and different decision makers typically see different portions of the cost. This may seem like a very abstract notion, so we will offer a simple example. An insurance plan wishes to increase use of a generic drug rather than the brand-name equivalent. The generic product costs a total of $50, of which $4 is paid by the patient and $46 is paid by the plan. The branded product costs a total of $100, of which $5 is paid by the patient and $95 is paid by the plan. From the plan's perspective, switching to the generic saves $49. From the consumer's perspective, switching to the generic saves $1. From the perspective of society as a whole, switching to the generic saves $50. These different perspectives are all valid, yet they may lead to very different choices.

Another example shows how differences in cost perspectives can lead to very different perceptions of the cost of a good or service. Suppose that the same HMO also encourages use of over-the-counter drugs because they are not a covered benefit. The over-the-counter product costs a total of $10, of which $0 is paid by the plan. The prescription product costs a total of $15, of which $5 is paid by the patient and $10 is paid by the plan. From the perspective of consumers, the switch to over-the-counter drugs increases costs from $5 to $10. Because consumers share the costs of covered medications with many other beneficiaries, they can be expected to want to switch to over-the-counter medications only if they are better (more effective or more convenient) than prescription medications. From the perspective of the insurer, the switch reduces costs from $10 to $0. The switch makes sense for the insurer as long as the prescription medication is not "too much better" than the over-the-counter medications. From the perspective of society, the switch reduces costs from $15 to $10. The switch makes sense only if the over-the-counter medication is "nearly as good" as the prescription medication.

A **societal perspective** on costs is usually the right perspective for two reasons. The societal perspective recognizes all costs, no matter to whom they accrue. For decisions involving the society as a whole, this is clearly the right perspective, and should be used by individuals, health plans, and providers as well. Other perspectives typically involve shifting costs to other parties, which is seldom a good long-run strategy. Those to whom costs have been shifted try to avoid them and try to avoid contracting with organizations that shift costs to them.

12.2.2 Identifying Resources and Opportunity Costs

Costs equal the volume of resources used in an activity multiplied by the opportunity cost of those resources. It is useful to keep these two components of cost separate, because either can vary between settings. A good clinical understanding of a process makes it easy to identify the resources used in an intervention; a well-documented clinical pathway makes it easier still.

Most of the time the opportunity cost of a resource simply equals what you paid for it. The opportunity cost of $100 in supplies is $100. The opportunity cost of an hour of nursing time is $27 if the total compensation of a nurse is $27 per hour. Things can get more complex when the cost of a resource has changed since you bought it or if you would no longer buy it at current prices. In those cases you have to calculate the value of the resource in its best alternative use, which can be a complicated process.

Economic theory gives us a powerful tool for simplifying cost analyses. It says, "Focus on the resources that you add (or do not need) as a result of this intervention." This is equivalent to saying, "Focus on incremental costs." Even this can be difficult, but one need not ponder exactly what proportion of the chief financial officer's compensation should be allocated to a triage process in the emergency room.

12.2.3 Direct and Indirect Costs

Implicit in this advice is a recommendation to focus on the direct costs of interventions. Direct costs result because an intervention has been tried. For example, the costs of a drug and its administration are direct costs of drug therapy. The costs of associated inpatient and outpatient care are also direct costs. If there are healthcare costs associated with ineffectiveness or adverse outcomes, those should be counted as well. By the same token, costs that the patient incurs because he or she undertakes this treatment are direct costs. Added child care, transportation, and dietary costs that result directly from therapy should be counted from a social cost perspective. If the perspective was that of the healthcare system, these added costs for patients would not be counted. (Of course, as we noted above, a cost perspective that ignores the effects on customers is likely to result in poor decisions.)

Most "indirect" costs represent a confusion of costs with benefits. Healthier people typically spend more on food, recreation, entertainment, and other joys of life, but this additional spending is not a part of the costs of interventions that restored health. (Individuals have independently made the judgment that this additional spending is worth it.) By the same token we should not treat a recovered patient's future spending as a cost of the intervention that permitted her recovery (unless, as with transplant patients' immunosuppressive drugs, those costs are an integral part of the intervention). That a transplant patient feels healthy enough to play tennis certainly signals that her operation was a success, but the cost of knee surgery for this overenthusiastic athlete should not be reckoned as a cost of the transplant.

12.3 Types of Analysis

We have identified four types of analysis: CBA, CEA, CUA, and CMA. The reader should be warned that mislabeling is the norm, not the exception. A "cost benefit analysis" could be anything, and the meaning of "cost-effectiveness analysis" has changed over the years. Figure 12.1 shows when each is needed.

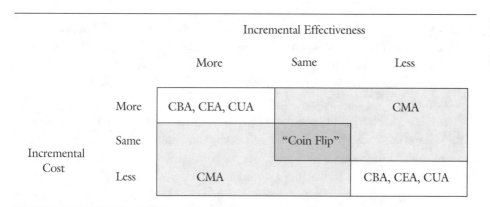

FIGURE 12.1
Using Decision
Support Tools

If it is really difficult to decide which strategy is best, then it shouldn't matter, since all of these techniques are designed to support decision making. If the options look so similar that it is hard to say which is best, do not do a detailed analysis. A "coin flip" will suffice. Of course, when populations are large, even small differences in cost or benefit per case can result in significant differences from society's perspective. However, for working managers, small differences are not worthy of attention.

12.4 CMA: Cost Minimization Analysis

The simplest and most productive type of analysis is CMA, which identifies the alternative with the lowest costs. As long as it has other outcomes at least as good as the other interventions, a CMA is the analysis of choice. While CMA is robust because it avoids most of the problems associated with measuring benefits, it does not do so entirely because there needs to be evidence that the interventions have comparable outcomes. The most common problem in CMA is a lack of evidence that the least-cost option has outcomes at least as good as the other choices.

Steps in CMA

1. Estimate the expected costs for each option.
2. Show that the least-cost option has outcomes at least as good as higher-cost alternatives.

A CMA Example

Which anesthesia strategy costs least for female patients undergoing abdominal surgery? Suver and his colleagues performed this CMA (without calling it a CMA) in an HMO hospital (1995). They compared use of propofol and a combination of tiopental and isoflurane. Recognizing that differences in the costs of acquiring and administering these anesthetics represented only part of the story, the team summarized preoperative, operative, recovery room, and ward costs for two small groups of patients. As you can see in Figure 12.2, propofol cost slightly less.

A concern about numbers like these is that they are based on what is commonly called *a full-resource cost accounting model*. That is to say, each cost center (e.g., preoperative) includes not only variable costs like labor and supplies, but also allocated fixed costs like the operating room equipment and general administration. At this point economists are fond of asking questions such as, "Would spending on operating room equipment or general administration change if we changed anesthetics?" Obviously not. Fortunately, looking just at consumables also suggests that using propofol reduces costs, although by about $48 per patient instead of $204.

Recall that, to be valid, a CMA needs to demonstrate that the less expensive strategy offers outcomes of care that are at least as good as the alternative. The analysts found no statistically significant differences in vital signs or outcomes. In addition, since propofol patients used less medication to prevent vomiting and reported fewer adverse events, it appears that propofol gives outcomes of care at least as good as thiopental/isoflurane. Therefore, while the savings (about $48 per patient in consumables) are modest, it is still a logical choice to switch to propofol as the standard anesthetic.

FIGURE 12.2

A Cost Minimization Analysis

	Propofol		Thiopental/Isoflurane	
	Allocated costs	Consumables	Allocated costs	Consumables
Preoperative	$11	$10	$12	$14
Operative	254	62	254	94
Recovery	180	39	180	47
Ward	1,159	45	1,312	49
	$1,604	$156	$1,758	$204

12.5 CEA: Cost-Effectiveness Analysis

CEA recognizes that it may be useful, when a more effective intervention costs more, to measure the incremental cost of improving outcomes. In at least some cases the incremental cost will be so high or so low that a decision can be made. In our detailed example below, CEA estimates the cost per life-year saved.

In some cases CEA is not helpful. If the cost per life-year saved is $35,000 or if the cost per injury prevented is $10,000, what to do will not seem obvious. In these cases CBA or CUA may be needed.

Steps in CEA

1. Estimate the expected costs for each option.
2. Establish how much the higher-cost option improves outcomes.
3. Calculate the cost per unit of improvement in outcome (e.g., the cost per life year gained or the cost per infection avoided).

A CEA Example

Is using a nicotine patch to help smokers quit cost-effective? It appears that it is. To do this cost-effectiveness calculation we need to know how much this intervention costs and how much it increases the percentage of smokers who quit smoking. The cost of the intervention depends on the cost of the additional counseling that is required, the cost of the patch itself, and how long the smoker will use it. The baseline estimate is that an eight-week treatment will cost $224 and five minutes of a physician's time will cost $11.64 (Wasley et al. 1997).

Patients who get the patch and counseling report a six-month quit rate of 22 percent. Patients who get only counseling report a six-month quit rate of 9 percent. This differential must be adjusted because about a third of patients will resume smoking, even after they have quit for a year, and some patients would have quit in the future even without the intervention. Compared to patients who get neither the patch nor counseling, the cost per additional quitter is $1,062. Compared to patients who get just counseling, the cost per additional quitter is $1,976. These costs are relatively high because most patients do not quit despite the intervention; some patients would have quit anyway; some patients relapse; and some patients do not use the patch, or use it ineffectively.

Stopping smoking has powerful effects on health, so the intervention looks very cost-effective. For a man aged 40 to 44, the cost per added year of life is only $993 to $1,847. For women of the same age, the cost per added year of life is only $1,770 to $3,293.

12.6 CBA: Cost Benefit Analysis

CBA is also relatively simple, but its validity is unknown. CBA is appropriate when the option with the best outcomes costs more. CBA begins with a comparison of two or more options to find out how their costs differ, then attempts to estimate the difference in benefits directly. There are two very different strategies for estimating benefits. One uses statistical techniques to infer how much consumers are willing to pay to avoid risks, the other uses surveys of the relevant population to determine whether the added benefits are worth the cost.

Neither method's validity has been clearly established. The fundamental challenge arises from concerns about consumers' abilities to make decisions involving small probabilities of harm. If consumers do not assess the probabilities correctly, their life choices and their responses to surveys are not likely to be reliable. In addition, there are always multiple challenges to the validity of statistical inferences, and statistical estimates of benefits are typically fairly imprecise. The problem with surveys is that they may not give us valid measures of "willingness to pay" or "willingness to accept compensation." First, consumers are often being asked to make complex assessments about services that they have not yet used. Answers to hypothetical, complex questions are suspect. Second, consumers may be inclined to misrepresent their preferences, believing that they will have to pay more out-of-pocket if they answer willingness-to-pay questions accurately. Therefore, even though CBA can provide invaluable information to decision makers, its accuracy can be suspect.

Steps in CBA

1. Estimate the expected incremental costs of the more expensive option.
2. Survey consumers to find out whether they would be (a) willing to pay enough to cover the added costs of an option with better outcomes or (b) willing to accept compensation that would be less than the cost savings of an option with worse outcomes.
3. Or, use market data to estimate how much consumers are willing to pay to avoid risks or willing to accept to take on risks.
4. Compare the incremental benefits and costs.

Two other complaints about CBA should be noted. Early CBA studies based estimates of benefits on estimates of increases in labor market earnings. A few minutes of reflection will tell you that there are problems with this approach. Is improved health for retired persons of no value? If people are willing to pay out-of-pocket for the care of their pets (who have no earning power), aren't changes in earnings a poor guide to the value of medical interventions? Earnings-based estimates of benefits have left a legacy of skepticism about CBA among healthcare analysts. A second complaint about CBA is that willingness to pay usually rises with income. This is profoundly troubling to analysts who would prefer a healthcare system that is more egalitarian than the current system in the United States. (While this is not really a criticism of CBA, it is sometimes presented as such.)

To illustrate how CBA works, return to the example of the switch from a branded product to a generic one. Recall that the branded drug cost $100 and the generic cost $50. An uninsured consumer would buy the branded product only if its benefits were large enough for her to be willing to pay $50. Few consumers would be willing to pay this much to get the branded product, because branded and generic products seldom differ. For existing users of a branded drug, however, there are both real and perceived risks of switching, such as risks of allergic reactions to differences in inert ingredients and risks of differences in therapeutic effectiveness due to differences in packaging. Remember, from the consumer's perspective, the cost differential is only $1, from $5 for the branded product to $4 for the generic. Current users of the drug may answer that they would be "willing to pay" $75, in which case the marginal benefit of the branded drug will appear to be larger than its marginal cost. Current users have an incentive to make sure that others bear the financial risks of higher costs. Asking people who are not current users is problematic as well. The opinion of someone who does not have a disease or has not used both drugs in question is not likely to hold much value.

A CBA Example

Do the benefits of poison control centers exceed their costs? A team from the University of California-San Francisco found that the average respondent was willing to pay just under $6 per month to have access to a poison control center (Phillips et al. 1997). This easily exceeded the cost of providing the services of a poison control center, which averaged less than 10 cents per household per month.

For several reasons, willingness to pay represents an attractive way of measuring the benefits of a service like a poison control center. First and foremost, both the caller and the victim typically benefit from the service. Even if the caller knows the victim only casually, it seems likely that he or she would be willing to pay something to reduce the stress and anxiety associated with a poisoning. Second, most of the benefits of a poison control center are intangible. Few poisonings result in serious injury or death, and most can be treated at home. Third, people may be willing to pay a little just to know that the service is there, even if they are not likely to use it.

The team elicited this information via a telephone survey of Bay Area residents. The sample included three groups. One group consisted of residents who had tried to call, but had been blocked from using the local poison control center because their county government refused to contribute its share of the budget. Less than one percent of this group was unwilling to pay anything for access. Another group consisted of residents who had called the poison control center. Again, under one percent of this group was unwilling to pay anything for access. A third group consisted of residents who had never called the poison control center, of which twenty percent was unwilling to pay anything for access.

Surveyors elicited willingness to pay data via a bidding process. They asked respondents whether they would be willing to pay a randomly chosen amount per month for access to the center. If the respondent said, "No," the surveyor countered with a lower number. If the respondent said, "Yes," the surveyor countered with a higher number.

Although the simplicity and power of these results demonstrates some of the attractions of a CBA, this study also points out some of the associated pitfalls. Responses were significantly influenced by the initial willingness to pay what surveyors suggested to them. The possibility that the interviewers, who already had an answer in mind, biased the study's results cannot be ruled out. In addition, the interviewers did not try to offer alternative uses of funds or get respondents to rank types of spending. Some studies have found that focusing on one service tends to inflate respondents' willingness to pay. Fundamentally, we still do not know how valid respondents' answers are, although it seems unlikely that the conclusions of this study are totally incorrect, given that willingness to pay was 50 times cost.

12.7 CUA: Cost Utility Analysis

CUA rivals CBA as a complete comparison of alternative interventions (note that a number of analysts do not distinguish between CEA and CUA). CUA seeks to measure consumer values by eliciting valuations of health states. This information is then used to "quality adjust" health gains, so that decision makers can consider the cost per quality-adjusted life year [QALY] saved (we will explain how QALYs are calculated later).

CUA is not simple and its validity is unknown. CUA is appropriate whenever CBA is, and at a formal level the two are essentially equivalent. At a practical level, however, the process of calculating benefits is different. CUA measures how alternative interventions change the health status of patients and how patients evaluate those changes.

Steps in CUA

1. Estimate the expected costs for each option.
2. Estimate the number of people alive in each year in each cohort.
3. Using a survey of consumers, estimate the average utility score for each option for each person who is alive in each year.
4. Multiply the utility score (which will range from zero to one) by the number of people alive in each year for all the cohorts being compared. The product is the number of Quality Adjusted Life Years (QALYs) for each cohort.
5. Discount the QALYs using rates of 2 to 5 percent.
6. Add the QALYs for each option, then find the difference.
7. Divide the difference in cost between options by the difference in QALYs.
8. Decide whether the cost per QALY is "too high."

Figure 12.3 walks through the calculations for a CUA. Suppose that 215 people each get treatments A and B. At the end of one year the number of survivors differs for the two treatments (N_A and N_B), as does the average utility level (U_A and U_B). We use these data to calculate how many additional QALYs we get as a result of using treatment B. We then calculate the cost per QALY if we switch to treatment B.

Four uncertainties are associated with this calculation, aside from the usual problems in assessing the clinical effectiveness of treatments. First, should we be limiting our questions to patients? Family, friends, and strangers sometimes are willing to help patients afford care. Second, can patients answer our questions about satisfaction adequately and accurately? Third, what discount rate should we use? While the example uses 3 percent, another rate might give us different answers, and we do not know what the right rate is. Fourth, assuming all other calculations are correct, at what cost per QALY should we draw the line? At the risk of sounding unduly negative, we note that the validity of CUA hinges on finding satisfactory answers to these questions, which is not likely.

Unlike CMA or CBA, CUA requires that the analyst explicitly discount future QALYs. A technique that is commonly used in banking and finance, **discounting** reflects that benefits that we realize far in the future are worth less than benefits we realize now. This is true because money can earn interest. As a result, to pay a bill that will come due in the future, one can set aside a smaller amount today. For example, if we invest $100 at an interest rate of 7 percent, we will have $160.58 at the end of ten years. We can also use this calculation to say that the value of a guaranteed payment of $160.58 that we will get in ten years is $100.

As long as the interest rate is fixed, the mathematics of discounting are easy to do on a spreadsheet. A single formula, $PV \times (1 + r)^n = FV$, lets us do all the calculations that we need to do. In this formula, PV refers to the "present value" of future costs or benefits, or the amount we are investing today; r refers to the interest rate; n refers to the number of time periods involved; and FV refers to the "future value" of future costs or benefits, or the amount we will have at the end of our investment. In discounting we use this same formula to calculate the present

	N_A	U_A	$N_A \times U_A$	N_B	U_B	$N_B \times U_B$	0%	3%
	QALY$_A$			QALY$_B$			QALY$_B$–QALY$_A$ discounted	
Year 1 outcomes	200	0.95	190.00	210	0.96	201.60	11.60	11.26
Year 2 outcomes	195	0.94	183.30	199	0.93	185.07	1.77	1.67
							13.37	12.93
Cost per QALY (with a $300,000 cost difference between A and B)							$22,438	$23,201

FIGURE 12.3
A Cost-Utility Analysis

value of future costs and benefits. The formula now becomes $PV = FV/(1 + r)^n$. If we knew the size and timing of an intervention's costs and benefits and if we knew the right discount rate, it would be a simple matter to calculate the present value of the QALYs associated with it. In fact, we don't know the right discount rate and we are not sure that the discount rate is constant for individuals, let alone the same for different individuals. Sensitivity analysis represents the best that we can do in this regard. This entails varying the discount rate over a "reasonable" range (typically 0 to 10 percent) and seeing if the answer changes. If not, the result is insensitive to the value of the discount rate that we use. But if the answer does change, we have to use our judgment.

A CUA Example

Are automobile air bags cost-effective? A highly skilled team from the Harvard Center for Risk Analysis studied this question, and concluded that the answer depended heavily on the location of the air bag (Graham et al. 1997). This study, unlike the nicotine patch example (Wasley et al. 1997), must confront the difficult issues posed by discounting and quality adjustment. The benefits of the study extend over a long period of time, and the authors chose to examine the cost per QALY, rather than the cost per death avoided.

The team began with baseline data about accidents, fatalities, non-fatal injuries, and seat belt use. They used this information to calculate the net number of deaths and injuries that would be avoided by use of air bags. (They looked at net deaths because, especially for infants, children, and very small adults, air bags can cause death in accidents that would not usually result in death.)

The team concluded that the incremental cost of equipping 10 million vehicles with driver's side air bags would be $2,210,000,000. They estimated that doing so would save 93,106 QALYs. As a result, the incremental cost-effectiveness ratio is just under $24,000 per QALY. At $1,331,000 the incremental cost of equipping 10 million vehicles with passenger's side air bags is substantially less. But, largely because front passenger seats are often unoccupied, the incremental effectiveness of air bags is much smaller. The team estimated that adding passenger's side air bags would save just 21,796 QALYs, meaning that the incremental cost per QALY was $61,000. Because a rule of thumb in CUA is that innovations are cost-effective if the cost per QALY is less than $50,000 and clearly not cost-effective if the cost per QALY is more than $100,000, passenger's side air bags are of uncertain value. There is strong support for the premise that the value of driver's side air bags exceeds their cost, as consumers in Asia and Europe are buying air bags voluntarily. Of course the inability of CUA to say whether passenger's side air bags are a good value or not is a shortcoming.

The study conducts a full-scale sensitivity analysis, in which the driver's side air bag remains cost-effective. Some of the changes in parameter push passenger's side air bags toward the cut-off point. For example, at the lower end of the effectiveness assumptions, the cost per QALY for passenger's side air bags exceeds $100,000.

To reinforce the point that many technical issues remain to be resolved in CUA, we note that this study includes the net change in healthcare costs as a part of the cost of air bags. This is controversial. We would argue that, although agreeing that a reduction in injuries is a benefit, this confuses two very separate decisions (whether to install air bags and how much medical care to seek, given crash-related injuries). Others would disagree. As always, the validity of the quality adjustment that underlies the construction of QALYs is unknown.

The real challenge, however, is to identify the options to which mandating air bags should be compared. For example, only when compared with stricter enforcement of seat belt laws or vigorous educational campaigns to encourage seat belt use can we really assess whether mandatory passenger's air bags are cost-effective.

12.8 Conclusion

Except for CMA or possibly a CEA, our advice is, "Don't try this at home." Where evidence is needed to make a decision, first turn to the literature. If no guidance is to be found there, do a CMA or CEA (or modify existing studies using your costs). If these tools do not provide a clear direction, use clinical judgement. CBA and CUA are research tools, not management tools.

Still, these techniques are useful in the process of making your organization more efficient. Applied judiciously, they will help your organization identify and provide the most efficient therapies, which will reduce your costs and increase your options.

Often lost in the discussion of these analyses is the importance of comparing the right options. Failing to compare reasonable alternatives renders CMA, CEA, CBA, and CUA useless. The best choice will usually be clear if the most plausible alternatives are compared. And if the best choice is not clear, then either choice may be appropriate.

References

Graham, J. D., K. M. Thompson, S. J. Goldie, M. Segui-Gomez, and M. C. Weinstein. 1997. "The Cost-Effectiveness of Air Bags by Seating Position." *Journal of the American Medical Association* 278 (17): 1418–24.

Phillips, K. A., R. K. Homan, H. S. Luft, D. H. Hiatt, D. R. Olson, T. E. Kearney, and S. E. Heard. 1997. "Willingness to Pay for Poison Control Centers." *Journal of Health Economics* 16 (3): 343–57.

Suver, J., S. R. Arikian, J. J. Doyle, S. W. Sweeney, and M. Hagan. 1995. "Use of Anesthesia Selection in Controlling Surgery Costs in an HMO Hospital." *Clinical Therapeutics* 17 (3): 561–71.

Wasley, M. A., S. E. McNagny, V. L. Phillips, and J. S. Ahluwalia. 1997. "The Cost-Effectiveness of the Nicotine Transdermal Patch for Smoking Cessation." *Preventive Medicine* 26 (2): 264–70.

REGULATION

Key Concepts

- Healthcare is extensively regulated.
- Regulation can make or break an organization (or its competitors).
- The explicit objective of regulation is consumer protection.
- The rationale for consumer protection regulations is consumer ignorance.
- Legislation and regulation reflect interest group politics.
- When markets are imperfect, regulation can only sometimes improve outcomes.
- Providers are likely to "capture" the regulatory process.
- Market responses to consumer ignorance can limit the need for regulation.

13.1 Introduction

Healthcare is extensively regulated, with new regulations constantly under consideration. This is important to managers for four reasons.

1. Changes in regulations can make or break an organization. For example, in 1998 the Health Care Financing Administration required that home healthcare firms obtain surety bonds to participate in Medicare. That this regulation was later rescinded did not help firms that went out of business because of it. In addition, regulations can be powerful competitive tools. Claims of regulatory violations by competitors can delay or derail projects, even if the claims are ultimately dismissed. Obviously, then, understanding the impact of regulations on one's organization, reacting effectively to changes in regulations, and knowing when political action is essential represent vital skills.

2. Managers need to understand the impetus behind healthcare regulation. Regulations are politically acceptable because the complexity of healthcare makes consumers feel vulnerable. Healthcare organizations must address these feelings of vulnerability, as failure to do so invites regulation or loss of business.

3. Managers need to understand that legislating and regulating are continuing political contests. For most organizations these are risky contests in which they have little to gain and much to lose. Only a few organizations can command the political power to win lasting advantages through the political process, but all organizations need to be alert to the threats that these contests pose.

4. Some regulations work very poorly because they conflict with powerful financial incentives. Many of the same incentives that reinforce or undermine regulations also affect private contracts. Understanding when regulations or contracts will achieve their goals is a necessary skill for managers.

It is important to understand that the choice is not between markets and regulation. Markets do not work without rules, and regulations do not work in isolation from market forces. The choice is between alternative sets of rules, and the stakes can be high.

13.2 Market Imperfections

Objections to regulation often stress that unfettered markets serve consumers well. This may be true for perfectly competitive markets, but most healthcare markets fall far short of this ideal. At the heart of these imperfections lies "rational consumer ignorance," which raises questions about the ability of consumers to make good choices. This is a very important issue in healthcare regulation, and we will discuss it in detail. Before doing so, however, we will briefly look at the three other main imperfections that healthcare markets suffer from: insurance, market power, and externalities.

13.2.1 Insurance

Insurance, by distorting consumers' incentives, reduces the likelihood that healthcare markets will be ideal. Patients are shielded from the true costs of healthcare, and even the most ethical provider will feel comfortable in recommending goods and services that the patient would be unwilling to buy if she faced the full cost. Moreover, the healthcare system in the United States also limits the role of consumers in choosing insurance plans. Because patients are so insulated from the true costs of care, it is unlikely that their healthcare choices reflect their values very well. This lack of connection between what consumers value and what healthcare products cost is an important market imperfection.

13.2.2 Market Power

Most healthcare providers have some market power, which means that prices will exceed marginal cost. To guarantee that markets will allocate resources at least as well as any other system, prices need to reflect the opportunity cost of using a good or service. By driving a wedge between the costs and prices of products, market power compounds the distortions introduced by insurance and may result in markets that do not function well. Moreover, market power means that price controls can be useful tools. In a perfectly competitive market, price controls can be irrelevant (when market prices fall below regulated levels) or harmful (when market prices rise above regulated levels). When there is significant market power, a third outcome is possible: price controls can result in lower prices and higher output. This does not mean that price controls are guaranteed to work in markets with significant market power—they can still be irrelevant or harmful. Rather, we mean to suggest that price controls can be beneficial if the distortions that they create are smaller than the distortions that they remove.

13.2.3 Externalities

Finally, some healthcare issues involve significant externalities. An **externality** is a benefit directly received by, or a cost directly imposed on, someone who is not a party to a transaction. For example, installation of a catalytic converter on a car in Los Angeles will make the air cleaner not only for the owner of the car, but others who live there and across the country as well. Markets tend not to work very well when there are significant externalities such as this. Consumers and producers generally focus on the private benefits of transactions, which results in underconsumption of products that generate external benefits, and overconsumption of products that generate external costs. Not surprisingly, the regulatory role of government tends to be substantial in these instances. For example, consider three activities that generate externalities: the search for new knowledge, the control of communicable diseases, or the maintenance of the environment. Patent and copyright laws restrict use of new knowledge, making it possible for its producers to profit from selling it, and encouraging production of it. Public health regulations can mandate immunizations or even require treatment of those who are infected with communicable diseases. Environmental regulations may restrict how resources are used or effectively change ownership rights. The details of these regulations can be quite controversial, but few societies leave resource allocation in such areas entirely to market forces.

13.3 Rational Consumer Ignorance

Healthcare regulations have multiple goals, but the ostensible objective of most regulations has long been consumer protection. The argument is that consumers need protection because they are rationally ignorant about the healthcare choices that they must make. Let us review why consumers are likely to be ignorant.

Healthcare choices are often difficult for anyone to make. In many cases decision makers have to rely on ambiguous or incomplete information. Although the scientific aura of modern medicine may suggest otherwise, a great many therapies lack a firm scientific basis. Even when the scientific evidence is good (in cases in which investigators have carried out controlled clinical trials), it may be difficult to apply to actual choices. It is often difficult to extrapolate from controlled trials to the uncontrolled environment of community practice, as the real world does not closely resemble a clinical trial. In any event, even valid evidence involves statements about probabilities, and most of us (including most healthcare providers) have difficulty using this sort of information well. We tend to see patterns where there are none, to overweight cases that are memorable or recent, and to ignore the rules of probability.

Patients face added problems in making healthcare decisions. To begin with, they often do not feel well and are experiencing a great deal of stress. Compounding this, they typically lack the experience, information, and skills that they need to make healthcare choices. Even after they have chosen a course of action, consumers may well have difficulty assessing whether the right diagnosis was made, the right therapy was chosen, or if that therapy was done properly.

The ignorance of most patients makes sense. Few of us know the healthcare choices that we will have to make or when we will have to make them, so we anticipate that the benefits of becoming well-informed are likely to be small and the costs are likely to be large. And even if we knew the choices that we would have to make, we would have difficulty forecasting our subsequent feelings. Left to our own devices, many of us would be flying blind. (Of course, rational ignorance is not universal. Patients with chronic illnesses often are quite well informed about their care because they may well have the time and the motivation to become knowledgeable.)

Struggling with such medical decisions makes consumers vulnerable in a number of ways. Consumers often do not know when to seek care. They can have difficulty evaluating the recommendations of healthcare professionals or the quality of care, as well as the actual price of that care. They may be unable to differentiate care that is worth more from care that simply costs more. To reduce their vulnerability, consumers may turn to medical professionals for advice.

Unfortunately, relying on provider recommendations does not end this vulnerability. Providers often have incentives to be imperfect agents. A provider may sell one product and not another, or one therapy may be much more profitable than another. In short, relying on providers for advice can reduce, but not necessarily end, consumers' vulnerability. In turn, they may react by using care that is not clearly beneficial or that is harmful, or by taking the advice of incompetent or unethical providers.

As a result, providers have an interest in reducing consumers' concerns about their vulnerability. Consumers who cannot distinguish good advice from bad may ignore all of it. Consumers who cannot distinguish reliable from unreliable healthcare professionals may patronize neither. Regulations can serve provider interests by sending a signal of quality to consumers. As long as competent, trustworthy professionals find it easier to live with the regulations than incompetent, untrustworthy professionals, regulations can be useful for both consumers and providers. Indeed, this is one reason why much of the demand for regulation comes from the groups to be regulated and why there is so much self regulation.

Rational ignorance, insurance-induced distortions, market-power-induced distortions, and externality-induced distortions mean that healthcare markets will be quite imperfect. This should not obscure an important fact: market imperfections do not guarantee that regulations will improve outcomes. Regulations are usually imperfectly designed and implemented as well. In addition, regulation's consumer-protection rationale may be just that: a rationale. Regulations can be used to gain a competitive advantage and may harm, not help, consumers.

Optometry Regulations

A study of optometry illustrates that regulations that are ostensibly designed to protect consumers can impose substantial costs on them (Haas-Wilson 1986). Recognizing that optometrists have better information about product quality and price than consumers, a number of states enacted restrictions on commercial practices, seemingly to prevent providers from taking advantage of consumers. These regulations prohibited employment of optometrists by nonprofessionals, limited the number and location of offices that optometrists could operate, and restricted use of trade names by optometrists who were employed by nonprofessionals. In essence, these regulations erected barriers to entry for chains by forcing them to operate more like solo practice optometrists.

These restrictions on chains appear to have increased the total price of glasses and examinations by 5–13 percent, with no apparent impact on quality. This conclusion is based on a statistical comparison of prices, the thoroughness of eye examinations, and the accuracy of prescriptions in regulated and unregulated states. The comparisons suggest that optometry regulations allowed one group of firms (solo optometrists) to use the regulatory process to gain a competitive advantage over another group of firms (chain optometries), with consumers losing as a result.

13.4 The Interest Group Model of Regulation

Legislation need not serve the public interest. Noting that groups can use regulations to expand their markets and gain market power, the **interest group model of regulation** argues that legislatures are similar to markets, in that individuals and groups seek regulations to further their interests. Indeed, regulatory barriers to competition are often better than other competitive advantages, because they are often harder for competitors to breach (especially for new firms or firms from outside the area, who will have little or no political influence). After all, product features can be duplicated and marketing plans can be copied by even the most insignificant start-up firm; but large, well-established firms have a significant advantage in the political arena.

13.4.1 Limiting Competition

One of the best ways to gain market power is to limit competition. Regulation is a very effective way of doing this. For example, when confronted by the challenge of freestanding ambulatory surgical centers, the American Hospital Association sought to use state Certificate of Need laws to restrict their expansion. Similarly, dental societies have long supported state laws making it illegal for persons not licensed as dentists to fit and dispense dentures. Note, however, that while lobbying the legislature to pass laws to prevent competition is perfectly legal, working together to prevent competition is illegal. In addition, the industry that is regulated is very likely to control the regulatory process, so the end result of consumer protection legislation may in fact represent "existing firm protection" and not the consumer at all. Managers need to understand that they cannot ignore politics—doing so can put an organization at risk.

13.4.2 Licensure

Licensing of healthcare professionals illustrates professional control of the regulatory process. Regulation of a profession can be done in a number of different ways. Quite often the type of regulation chosen protects the economic interests of the regulated group far better than it protects the health and safety interests of the public. States generally regulate health professionals via licensure, certification, and registration. Licensure makes it illegal to perform the duties of a profession without meeting requirements set by the state. Certification prohibits those who do not meet requirements set by the state from using a title, but not from practicing. Registration requires practitioners to file their names, addresses, and relevant qualifications.

Licensure is the most restrictive form of regulation. It can prohibit practice by individuals without the right qualifications or require that they practice under the supervision of another professional. Its use is often justified by concerns about safety. While recognizing that certification considerably reduces consumer ignorance, advocates of licensure contend that it does not prevent unwary consumers from making unsafe choices. This may be so, but licensure can also prevent consumers from making choices that might make sense for them. It forces consumers to use highly trained, very expensive personnel when there may be viable alternatives. As such, it represents a powerful weapon in the struggle with competing professional groups.

Lay Midwifery

A look at lay midwifery shows why this debate matters. A lay midwife typically enters the profession via independent midwifery school or apprenticeship, so she has substantially less training than a physician or a professional nurse-midwife. Thirty-six states restrict or prohibit the practice of lay midwifery and many hospitals will not grant privileges to professionals who assist in home deliveries. While safety concerns are usually cited as the prime motive, there is little actual evidence that such concerns are valid. In fact, the evidence suggests that death rates and complication rates are substantially lower in systems that make extensive use of lay midwives. For example, in the Netherlands, where roughly a third of births are home deliveries attended by lay midwives, death and complication rates are well below those of the United States (Hafner-Eaton and Pearce 1994). The historical record also suggests that quality concerns represent more of a smokescreen than a valid concern. Regulations limiting or prohibiting midwifery were enacted more than 100 years ago, when birth outcomes were clearly better for midwives than for physicians (apparently because midwives usually washed their hands as they moved between patients).

If the scientific evidence for banning midwives is not strong, the economic evidence for doing so is compelling (at least from the perspective of competing professional groups). The average cost of a birth assisted by a lay midwife is well below the cost of a birth assisted by a physician or nurse midwife. As a result, lay midwives could claim a significant share of the market, if only as a strategy for improving birth outcomes for under-served populations. Assuming for the moment that uncomplicated hospital-based births managed by highly trained healthcare professionals are safer, will women who cannot afford or prefer not to use hospital-based care be better off if that is their only choice? Even successful efforts to improve quality can harm consumers if the choice is between services of the highest quality and no services at all.

13.4.3 Regulation as a Competitive Strategy

Regulations typically increase a firm's costs and reduce its flexibility. A rule that affects the structure or process of an organization's operations can have no effect or it can increase costs. Naturally enough, firms seek to resist regulations (even if their business plans are consistent with the goals of the regulation). Of course, hamstringing rivals by imposing regulations on them (but not on oneself) can be a very effective competitive strategy. In fact, most regulation of the health professions has been a result of this strategy, because existing professionals have been "grandfathered" in, so that regulations apply only to newly licensed practitioners.

13.5 Regulatory Imperfections

When markets are not perfect, regulation can improve outcomes. For three reasons, however, regulation is likely to be imperfect as well: the need for decentralized decision making, conflicts between regulatory and financial incentives, and capture by the firms who are regulated.

Regulations work best when decision making is centralized and when "one size fits all." This is not the case in healthcare. Patients' healthcare needs, preferences, and circumstances vary considerably, so decision making needs to be decentralized and individualized. This limits the acceptable scope of regulations. In addition, regulatory and financial incentives need to be aligned to work well. Where this is not true, regulations are likely to be ignored or circumvented. For example, if it is more convenient for physicians to treat patients in the hospital than in their offices and there are no financial incentives to encourage outpatient care, utilization review is unlikely to reduce hospitalization rates. If we have learned anything during the last fifty years, we have learned that healthcare organizations respond to financial incentives.

Furthermore, the groups being regulated are likely to "capture" regulations based on even the most noble of intentions. Capture occurs when a group gains effective control of the administration of the regulations. Capture matters because how the laws are implemented and enforced is at least as important as the laws themselves, and sooner or later the groups being regulated are likely to take control of the enforcement process. They will have better information then consumers, will pay more attention to the regulatory process than consumers, and will have a more intense interest in the regulatory process than consumers. Regulation does not end the rational ignorance of consumers (although regulations that disclose information may reduce it). As a result, regulators are likely to be members of the regulated group or are likely to rely on members of the regulated group for advice. Compounding this dependence is the continuing interest in the regulations by the group being regulated. Consumers and their advocates, in contrast, are likely to lose interest once the problems that led to the regulations have eased. Finally, the group being regulated typically has an intense interest in the outcome of the process, and most consumers do not. This further increases the odds of capture, because in the political arena a small group with an intense interest is likely to prevail in a contest with a larger group with more diffuse interests. As a result, regulation can best be described as "for the profession" rather than "of the profession."

Self-Regulation

State regulation of the professions usually gives legal force to self-regulation by the profession. For example, according to the National Association of Boards of Pharmacy, state pharmacy boards have between 0 and 5 public members (Conlan 1997). Pharmacists represent a majority of the members of the board in every state. Not surprisingly, most pharmacists support state regulation of their profession and favor changes in the regulations that would appear to benefit pharmacists, not protect consumers.

A recent survey of pharmacists found that most were strongly opposed to periodic competency examinations. Evidently concerns that existing continuing education requirements have no "teeth" were outweighed by concerns that some pharmacists would be denied licenses. In contrast, the pharmacists surveyed favored increased regulation of mail order firms (which use equipment to dispense large volumes of chronic-care medications), ostensibly because they inadequately counsel patients. (That mail-order firms are formidable competitors, because they offer consumers convenience and low prices, was never mentioned as a concern.) At the same time, support for efforts to assess pharmacists' counseling efforts by state boards was weak.

This is a fairly typical example of a self-regulating profession that has been given state power to enforce its edicts. Not surprisingly, the interests of pharmacists appear to get priority over the interests of consumers.

As this example suggests, visions of ideal markets and ideal regulatory scenes are not very enlightening. Most healthcare markets are imperfect, as are most healthcare regulations. Whether regulating markets or deregulating markets will best serve consumers is an empirical question.

13.6 Market Responses to Market Imperfections

Market responses to consumer ignorance can limit the need for regulation. Even imperfectly functioning markets incorporate incentives to serve consumers well. For most providers, repeat sales and customers are essential, so the incentives to meet customers' expectations are strong. Even when repeat customers may not be a major part of the business (as with a nursing home or plastic surgeon), the provider's reputation usually represents one of its most important assets. Only when customers are not likely to detect poor performance are agency problems apt to be profound. Because consumers are often aware of their ignorance and know they may have difficulty assessing poor performance, they are willing to pay for information about quality and turn to consumer organizations (such as the American Association of Retired Persons) or information services (such as the National Committee for Quality Assurance) to aid them. These market responses will not eliminate all the imperfections in healthcare markets, but they do remind us that flawed markets need not be worse than flawed regulations.

13.6.1 Tort and Contract Law

Tort law (which addresses compensation for a broad array of injuries) and contract law (which addresses failure to keep agreements) can also remediate the shortcomings of healthcare markets, and these legal remedies have some powerful advantages. First, the threat of action is often enough to ensure compliance with explicit or implicit norms. If the probability of detecting noncompliance is high enough and the penalties are large enough, legal action may be uncommon. Second, unless the expected cost of performance exceeds an agent's financial liability for nonperformance, tort and contract law create incentive for providers to perform. Legal liability can result in legal costs, fines and penalties, and damage to one's reputation, all of which agents will want to avoid. Third, legal liability is outcomes oriented. Historically, regulation has focused on whether the structure of care and the processes of care comply with unverified norms. Obviously, the utility of this is limited. Fourth, the legal system is more difficult to "capture" than most regulatory systems, especially when plaintiffs can take their cases to juries. Because consumers can initiate legal action themselves and because some lawyers are willing to accept the financial risks of failed suits by accepting contingency fees, access to legal remedies is more difficult to restrict than regulatory remedies. (Although the "tort reforms" of the last decade had this as an objective.)

There are disadvantages to tort and contract law. To begin with, legal remedies are costly to apply. Typically, because of the costs of bringing suit, consumers may face barriers in accessing the legal system. And of course, consumer ignorance may compromise the effectiveness of legal remedies. If consumers do not realize that their bad outcome is due to a breach of duty on the part of their provider, they will not bring suit. Alternatively, ignorant consumers may file suits when undesired outcomes are due to bad luck, not negligence. These problems can sharply reduce the effectiveness of the legal system. Absent a credible threat of being sued, incompetent or unscrupulous providers can continue unchecked. Even worse, the incentive for competent, scrupulous providers to invest resources in improving the quality of care may be diluted.

13.6.2 Information Dissemination

Two examples illustrate both the power and limits of the legal system. First, the legal system has limited physicians to areas in which they are competent, even more effectively than state licensing boards. Medical licenses do not recognize differences in the skills of physicians. Were licenses the only guide, family practitioners would be able to perform neurosurgery. In fact, the threat of liability claims leads hospitals to limit practices of physicians and physicians to restrict their practices.

A second and less happy story emerges from studies of medical malpractice. It appears that the overwhelming majority of consumers who have suffered serious injuries as a result of negligence do not sue and receive no compensation. In addition, a high proportion of malpractice suits does not appear to involve provider negligence (Weiler et al. 1993). As a result, no one gets very useful information about quality from the malpractice system, and it is not clear that malpractice litigation has improved the quality of care. In principle, publication of providers' malpractice histories might help consumers choose. Better yet, publication of risk-adjusted outcomes data would put pressure on organizations to improve quality, and could reduce consumer ignorance as well.

Regulations Can Change Consumer Information

Regulations can, of course, seek to offer consumers information instead of "protecting" them from the consequences of their ignorance. For example, in the late 1980s the New York State Department of Health began sharing heart surgery mortality rates with hospitals. (To the extent possible, these rates were adjusted for differences in the risk of death that hospitals and physicians could not control.) Covering individual surgeons as well as hospitals, the ratings were initially given only to hospitals, but court rulings forced the Department to publish its data. Since the publication of the information, crude mortality rates have fallen by more than 20 percent and risk-adjusted mortality rates have fallen by more than 40 percent. Much of this appears to be a result of consumers seeking care from providers with low mortality rates. Both surgeons and hospitals with above-average outcomes appear to have gained market share since the rankings have been made public (Mukamel and Mushlin 1998).

It is an open question whether information release must be mandatory. Both the New York example and the National Practitioner Data Bank (which assembles data disciplinary actions against physicians) are mandatory, but information dissemination appears to be taking on a life of its own. Not only have managed care organizations started moving toward a structured release of information via the Health Plan and Employer Data and Information Set, but larger purchasers and purchaser coalitions are beginning to ask for data. For example, the Cleveland Health Quality Choice Program publishes data on length of stay, mortality rates, and patient satisfaction. If the market demands information, providers will furnish it.

13.6.3 Contracts

Contracts represent a private regulatory system (albeit one that will not work if a collective mechanism for enforcing contracts does not function effectively). As with public regulations, contracts work best when financial and regulatory incentives are aligned. A contract that pays more for better performance will usually provide more satisfactory results than a contract that stipulates what is minimally acceptable.

For example, modifying physicians' practice patterns represents a central challenge for physician organizations. Robinson (1999) notes that, under a pure capitation contract, physicians have financial incentives to avoid chronically ill patients, not to provide some types of care, and to refer large numbers of patients to other providers. Under a pure fee-for-service contract, in contrast, physicians have financial incentives to provide high volumes of billable services. Unfortunately, fee-for-service contracts also appear to result in fragmentation of care, upcoding, unbundling, and provision of services of questionable clinical value.

The response of a number of large practice organizations has been to set up contracts with physicians that blend capitation and fee-for-service payment. These contracts combine risk-adjusted capitation for basic primary care services, capitation stop-loss provisions to protect physicians from unexpectedly high costs, and fee-for-service payments for targeted services. These targeted services include vaccinations, visits to nursing facilities, and services entailing expensive supplies. The contracts also offer higher capitation rates for providers who provide a broader range of services. These contracts seek to change practice patterns by aligning the incentives of the organization and the physicians.

13.7 Implications for Managers

The choice is not between markets or regulation, because without regulation, markets will perform poorly and may not exist. The choice is between alternative regulatory systems.

Healthcare managers must understand the importance of regulations for their organizations and incorporate the effects of regulations in their decision making. Losses in the legislative or bureaucratic arenas may result in regulations that put an organization at a significant disadvantage. Although it is tempting to see regulations as competitive tools, in practice their value is usually limited in competing with rivals in the same sector. Although zoning laws and Certificate of Need laws are notable exceptions, regulations usually apply the same rules for all the competitors in a sector.

Even when regulations could afford them a competitive advantage (perhaps by suppressing competition from rivals from other sectors), few organizations have the political strength and staying power to secure a long-lasting competitive advantage through political action. The exceptions tend to be large, have a well-defined goal that their members share, are well-funded, have a positive image in the eyes of the public, and appear to be advocating policies that benefit the wider public. (Of course, less influential interest groups often have the capacity to shape laws and the subsequent regulations when the stakes are small for other groups.) For most organizations the challenge will be to resist legislation and administrative rulings that threaten to put them at a disadvantage. Fortunately, preventing change usually takes much less influence than does causing it.

In fact, the interests of healthcare providers appear to require more regulation than governments can be induced to provide. Non-governmental regulation is widespread in healthcare. For example, certification of health plans and physicians grew out of needs to give customers more detailed information about quality than regulatory bodies could provide. This trend is likely to continue. Managers need to prepare their organizations to compete in environments in which competitive pressures force the release of detailed, audited information about costs and outcomes. Organizations that cannot attract well-informed customers are likely to fail.

13.8 Conclusion

Markets and regulations are not competing strategies. Markets need a sound regulatory underpinning to work. These underpinnings need to secure property rights, define liability, create a mechanism for enforcing contracts, and establish what forms of competition are permitted. For example, Enthoven and Singer (1997) point out that an effectively functioning insurance market requires an efficient mechanism for deciding when care is "medically necessary." Such a mechanism benefits both insurers and patients. Too much ambiguity will depress sales of insurance, because consumers will perceive that their contract's promises are essentially meaningless. On the other hand, simple, rigid interpretations of "medically necessary" will ignore the diverse circumstances that consumers face, or will allow costs to skyrocket. Designing effective regulations is not easy. Even well-intentioned regulations can stifle innovation, and there is no guarantee that regulations will be well-intentioned.

References

Brennan, T. A., and D. M. Berwick. 1966. *New Rules: Regulation, Markets, and the Quality of American Health Care*. San Francisco: Jossey-Bass, 205.

Conlan, M. F. 1997. "Board Games: Many R.Ph.s are Unclear over State Pharmacy Boards' Missions." *Drug Topics* 141(22): 58–63.

Enthoven, A. C, and S. J. Singer. 1997. "Markets and Collective Action in Regulating Managed Care." *Health Affairs* 16 (6): 26–32.

Haas-Wilson, D. 1986. "The Effect of Commercial Practice Restrictions: The Case of Optometry." *Journal of Law and Economics* 24, 165–84.

Hafner-Eaton, C., and L. K. Pearce. 1994. "Birth Choices, the Law, and Medicine: Balancing Individual Freedoms and the Protection of the Public's Health." *Journal of Health Politics, Policy and Law* 19 (4): 813–35.

Mukamel, D. B., and A. I. Mushlin. 1998. "Quality of Care Information Makes a Difference: An Analysis of Market Share and Price Changes after Publication of the New York State Cardiac Surgery Mortality Reports." *Medical Care* 36 (7): 945–54.

Robinson, J. C. 1999. "Blended Payment Methods in Physician Organizations Under Managed Care." *Journal of the American Medical Association* 282 (13): 1258–63.

Weiler, P. C., H. H. Hiatt, J. P. Newhouse, W. G. Johnson, T. A. Brennan, and L. L. Leape. 1993. *A Measure of Malpractice: Medical Injury, Malpractice Litigation, and Patient Compensation*. Cambridge, MA: Harvard University Press.

PROFITS, MARKET STRUCTURE, AND MARKET POWER

Key Concepts

- If the demand for its products is not perfectly elastic, a firm has some market power.
- Most healthcare organizations have some market power because their rivals' products are not perfect substitutes.
- Having fewer rivals increases market power.
- Firms with no rivals are called **monopolists**; firms with only a few rivals are called **oligopolists**.
- More market power allows larger markups over marginal cost.
- Barriers to entry increase market power.
- Regulation is often a source of market power.
- Product differentiation and advertising can also be sources of market power.

14.1 Introduction

What distinguishes very competitive markets (ones with below-average profit margins) from less competitive markets (ones with above-average profit margins)? An influential analysis by Michael E. Porter (1985) argues that profitability depends on five factors:

1. the nature of rivalry among existing firms,
2. the risk of entry by potential rivals,
3. the bargaining power of customers,
4. the bargaining power of suppliers, and
5. the threat from substitute products.

For the most part, Porter's model explains variations in profits in terms of variations in market power. Firms in industries with muted price competition, little risk of entry, limited customer bargaining power, and few satisfactory substitutes have a significant amount of market power. When firms have market power they face customer demands that are not particularly price elastic. As a result, markups can be large. We will use the Porter framework to examine the links between profits, market structure, and market power.

    Three characteristics of healthcare markets still tend to reduce their competitiveness. First, the structure of most healthcare markets has tended to mute rivalry among existing firms, since many have only a few competitors. Second, this muted rivalry persists in many healthcare markets because a broad array of cost and regulatory barriers limit entry. In many of these markets, new competitors, who would be tempted to compete on the basis of value to gain market share, are effectively barred. Third, there are relatively few close substitutes for many healthcare products. This makes the market demand less elastic and may make the demand for an individual firm's products less elastic. All of these factors tend to give healthcare firms market power and allow high markups.

The bargaining power of suppliers varies considerably. Some suppliers have very strong positions, while others do not. Although a detailed examination of differences in suppliers' bargaining power is beyond the scope of this book, one change is important to note. Physicians are suppliers to many healthcare organizations, and physicians' incomes have stagnated since the early 1990s. Their bargaining position has clearly deteriorated in recent years.

Unquestionably the most significant change in healthcare markets has been the growth of managed care. Managed care dramatically enhances the bargaining power of most healthcare customers. As a result, many healthcare firms face much more competitive markets and narrower margins than they are accustomed to.

Although it does not serve their customers well, profit-oriented managers will usually seek to gain market power. The most ambitious will try to change the nature of competition. For example, faced with determined managed care negotiators, healthcare providers have merged to reduce costs and to improve their bargaining positions. Both can substantially improve margins. But even when an organization cannot change the competitive structure of a market, it still has two options: it can seek to become the low-cost producer, or it can seek to differentiate its products from those of the competition. Either of those two strategies can boost margins, even in relatively competitive markets.

14.2 Rivalry Among Existing Firms

Most healthcare organizations have some market power, facing price elasticities of demand that are "small enough" so that they will not lose all of their business if their prices are a little higher than some rivals. Having market power has several implications. Obviously, it means that firms have some discretion on pricing since the market does not dictate what they will charge. Perhaps, less obviously, the prospect of market power also gives healthcare organizations a strong incentive to try to differentiate their products. Typically, the amount of market power an organization has depends on how successfully it can make the case that its products differ in terms of quality, convenience, or some other attribute, making product differentiation an important tool in the quest for market power.

The combination of flexibility in pricing and in product specifications makes managing an organization with market power (or hopes thereof) complex, because managers have to consider a broad range of strategies, including how to compete. In some markets there is aggressive price competition and competition in product innovation; in other markets there is not. Managers have to decide what the best strategy will be in their circumstances.

Healthcare organizations generally have market power because their competitors' products are *imperfect substitutes*. This can be true because of differences in location, in other attributes, or even in familiarity. For example, a pharmacy across town is less convenient than one nearby, even if it has lower prices. Because consumers choose to patronize the more expensive, but closer, pharmacy, it has some market power.

In addition, medical goods and services are typically "experience" products, in that consumers must use a product to ascertain that it offers better value than another. For instance, a patient must visit a new dentist who has just joined her dental plan to be sure that her needs will be met. Likewise, consumers will have to try a generic drug to be sure that it works as well as the branded version. Because of this need to try out healthcare products, it is costly to compare medical goods and services, and consumers tend not to change products when price differences are small. All of these factors make it more difficult to assess whether competing products are good substitutes, thus increasing market power.

As we will see in Section 14.7, decisions about advertising tend to be quite different when market power is based on differences in attributes rather than differences in information. Attribute-based differences usually demand extensive advertising. Information-based differences often reward restrictions on advertising.

In addition, many healthcare providers have a limited number of competitors. This is true for hospitals and nursing homes in most markets, and often for rural physicians. Whenever the market is small, either because the population is small or because the service is highly specialized, the number of competitors will usually be small. And when there are only a few rivals, all have some market power, if only because each controls a significant share of the market. With only a few competitors, firms recognize that they have some flexibility in pricing and that what their rivals do will affect them. Having a limited number of rivals results in market power.

Do physicians really have market power?

There appears to be fairly good evidence that they do, even though there are many physicians in most markets. Two studies have attempted to calculate the price elasticity of demand faced by individual physicians (Lee and Hadley 1981; McCarthy 1985). One estimated that physicians faced price elasticities on the order of -2.8 to -5.1; another found a very similar range of -3.1 to -3.3. Not surprisingly, the demand for the services of individual physicians is much more elastic than the demand for physicians' services as a whole. (After all, other physicians may not be perfect substitutes for your physician, but they are fairly close substitutes.) These elasticity estimates suggest that markups will be quite large, meaning that physicians have a good deal of market power.

Market conditions under perfect competition offer a baseline with which to contrast other market structures. No allocation system can be more efficient than a perfectly competitive market, in which buyers and sellers are price takers. That is to say, firms operate on the assumption that demand is very price elastic. The only way to realize above-normal profits is to be more efficient than the competition. Firms pay no particular attention to the actions of their rivals, in part because potential entrants face no barriers and in part because there are so many rivals. Organizations that face any other market structure will produce somewhat less and charge somewhat higher prices.

Few healthcare markets even remotely resemble perfectly competitive markets. A few markets have only one supplier and are said to be **monopolistic**. For example, the only pharmacist in town has a monopoly. A number of markets have many rivals, all claiming a small share of the market. At first glance these markets may look perfectly competitive, but there is one key difference: customers do not view the services of one supplier as perfect substitutes for the services of another. For example, one dentist might have a different location than another, a different personality, or a different treatment style. Markets like these are said to be **monopolistically competitive**.

Other markets have only a few competitors. These markets are said to be **oligopolistic**. Markets with many competitors can also be oligopolistic if a few competitors have a significant market share. A local market with two hospitals serving the same area is oligopolistic, as is a PPO market with 15 firms when the two largest firms have 40 percent of the market. Because the decisions of some competitors determine the best strategies of other rivals, oligopoly markets differ from other markets in an important way. Oligopolists must act strategically and recognize their mutual interdependence. We will explore this in more detail in Chapter 15.

14.3 Customers' Bargaining Power

A distinguishing feature of healthcare markets has long been that there are many buyers, all with limited bargaining power. This is no longer true. The emergence of managed care firms, which seek to identify efficient providers and those who will give substantial price concessions, changes the picture. (Of course, Medicare and Medicaid, the original PPOs, have had a major influence on healthcare markets since their inception.) So, in addition to the number of sellers, healthcare market structures depend on the market share of PPOs, of HMOs (in both instances including the market share of Medicare and Medicaid, where appropriate), and the number of each in the market.

Managed Care Affects Rivalry

By emphasizing price competition, the expansion of managed care appears to be changing the nature of rivalry in healthcare markets. A recent study of hospital costs reinforces this conclusion (Bamezai et al. 1999). Between 1989 and 1994, hospital costs grew much more slowly in markets with high HMO or PPO penetration than in markets with low penetration. Most of this difference appears to be due to the success of HMO and PPO plans in markets with keen competition among hospitals. In markets with more muted hospital competition, the impact of managed care has been much smaller. In markets with only a few hospitals or with a dominant system, managed care has done little to slow cost growth. Conversely, in markets with many competing hospitals, cost growth has not slowed unless managed care has successfully penetrated the market.

The study also supports the conjecture that HMOs do more to control costs than PPOs. In competitive, high-HMO markets, costs rose much more slowly than in competitive, high-PPO markets. This makes sense because HMOs usually build smaller provider networks than PPOs, so HMOs can be much more effective bargainers than PPOs. In addition, HMOs make more use of capitation and case rates, giving hospitals and physicians much stronger incentives to control costs.

These results suggest that HMOs are likely to become the dominant form of insurance in most markets. Unless consumers strongly prefer PPOs to HMOs, the emerging HMO cost advantage would seem to be a powerful marketing tool.

14.4 Entry by Potential Rivals

Barriers to entry often reduce the number of rivals in healthcare markets and may be market-based or regulation-based. Generally, regulation-based barriers are more effective. Whatever the source, restrictions on entry reduce the number of competing providers and make demand less price elastic. In other words, restrictions on entry increase market power, whether the restrictions are necessary or not.

The best way to erect entry barriers and gain market power is to have the government do it for you. This has two fundamental advantages. First, it is perfectly legal and eliminates public and private suits alleging antitrust violations. Second, this strategy usually creates market power more permanently, because entry barriers that do not have government sanction will usually be eroded by market competition or legal action.

State licensure forms much of the basis for market power in healthcare. Licensure can be used to prevent entry by suppliers with similar qualifications and to prevent encroachments by suppliers with lesser qualifications. For example, state licensure laws typically require that pharmacy technicians work under the direct supervision of registered pharmacists and that a registered pharmacist supervise no more than two technicians. While not very closely connected to the regulatory goal of reducing medication errors, these restrictions clearly protect jobs for pharmacists by limiting what technicians can do and limit encroachment by firms using automated dispensing equipment (operated by technicians).

Some entry barriers represent rewards for intellectual property rights. For example, innovating organizations can establish a monopoly for a limited period by securing patents. In the United States, patents give the holder a monopoly for 17 years. The patent holder must disclose the details of the new product or process in the application, but is free to exploit the patent and sell or license the patent rights. Patents are vitally important in the pharmaceutical industry, as generic products are excluded from the market until the patent expires.

Copyrights also create monopolies to protect intellectual property rights. Unlike patents, copyrights protect only a particular expression of an idea, not the idea itself. Copyright monopolies normally last for the life of the author plus 50 years. Trademarks (distinctive visual images that belong to a particular organization) also grant monopoly rights. As long as they are used and defended, trademarks never expire. All of these legal monopolies create formidable barriers to entry for potential competitors.

Strategic actions can also prevent or slow entry by rivals. Rivals will not want to launch unprofitable ventures, and firms can try to ensure that entrants will lose money. Preemption, limit pricing, innovation, and mergers are commonly used tactics. **Preemption** involves moving quickly to build excess capacity in a region or product line and ward off entry. For example, building a hospital that has excess capacity means that a second hospital would face formidable barriers. Not only would it exacerbate the excess capacity, but it could anticipate that this excess capacity would result in a price war. Managed care firms would not miss the opportunity to grab larger discounts. Worse still for the prospective entrant, most of the costs of the established firm are fixed costs. The established firm's incremental costs will be low, and its best strategy will be to capture as much of the market as it can by aggressive price cutting. For the rival, in contrast, all of its costs are incremental. It can avoid years of losses by building elsewhere.

Limit pricing is another tactic that established firms or those with established products can use. **Limit pricing** entails setting prices low enough to discourage potential entrants. It involves the calculation that, by giving up some profits now, the organization can prevent entry and avoid even bigger profit reductions later. (In essence, the firm acts as though demand were more elastic than it seems to be.) Limit pricing only works if the firm is an aggressive innovator. Otherwise, competitors will eventually be able to enter the market with lower costs or better quality, and the payoff to limit pricing will be minimal.

Innovation by established organizations can deter entry as well. Relentlessly reducing costs and improving quality means that entrants will always have to play catch-up, which does not promise substantial profits.

Mergers increase market power by changing market structure. A well-conceived, well-executed merger can reduce costs or increase market power, either of which can increase profit margins. (Of course many, perhaps most, mergers do not succeed because of failures in either conception or execution.) In principle, most mergers are consummated in the expectation that cost reductions will result from consolidation of some functions. Usually left unsaid in merger announcements is the anticipated improvement in the firm's bargaining position. Customers and suppliers usually must do business with the most important firms in a market. For example, failing to contract with a dominant health plan or health system will pose problems for their customers and suppliers, so larger firms anticipate getting better deals. Whether cost savings or market share gains are more important is controversial.

Mergers Result in Price Increases

A recent study of California hospitals during the years 1986 through 1994 implies that mergers among for-profit hospitals resulted in price increases ranging from 14.5 to 16.2 percent (Keeler et al. 1999). The study also implies that mergers among not-for-profit hospitals resulted in price increases ranging 0.3 to 7.3 percent. Of course the effects of mergers depend on the nature of the hospitals and the nature of competition. The study's estimates imply that if two small hospitals in a competitive metropolitan area merge, their ability to negotiate higher prices will be quite limited. In contrast, if two large hospitals in a smaller town merge, their ability to negotiate higher prices can be substantial.

   Another recent analysis finds that small hospitals can realize significant cost savings as a result of merging (Dranove 1998). It estimates that administrative costs per discharge are 34 percent lower in a 200-bed hospital than in a 100-bed hospital. Overall, cost per discharge in non-revenue cost centers is 24 percent lower in a 200-bed hospital than in a 100-bed hospital. For larger hospitals, in contrast, size conveys few cost advantages. Cost per discharge in non-revenue cost centers is only one percent lower in a 400-bed hospital than in a 200-bed hospital. Hence, the policy of the Federal Trade Commission and the Department of Justice not to challenge mergers if one of the hospitals has fewer than 100 beds appears to be a solid one. For small hospitals, mergers appear to promise lower costs. Of course, the evidence also supports the conclusion that mergers increase market power, therefore increasing profit margins.

14.5 Market Structure and Markups

Having market power does not change the rules for setting profit-maximizing prices. Organizations should still set prices so that marginal revenue equals its

FIGURE 14.1
Market Share and
Markups

Market share	Market elasticity	Firm's elasticity	Incremental cost	Profit maximizing price
48%	−0.60	−1.25	$10.00	$50.00
24%	−0.60	−2.50	$10.00	$16.67
7.5%	−0.60	−8.00	$10.00	$11.43
5%	−0.60	−12.00	$10.00	$10.91

This figure assumes that the firm's price elasticity equals the market elasticity divided by the firm's market share, which need not always be true.

marginal cost. And, of course, if the return on equity is not adequate, the organization should exit the line of business.

What does change are markups. A firm with substantial market power will find it profitable to set prices well above marginal cost. For example, Figure 14.1 shows that a firm with a substantial amount of market power ($\varepsilon = -2.5$) will have a 67 percent markup. In contrast, a firm with a moderate amount of market power ($\varepsilon = -8.0$) will only have a 14 percent markup. Finally, a firm with very little market power ($\varepsilon = -12.0$) will have a 9 percent markup.

Organizations with market power benefit from markup, but their customers do not; in fact, they will face higher prices, which in turn results in their using the product less, or not benefiting from it at all.

As a result, the goals of managers depend on whether they are buying or selling. Managers seek to reduce the market power of their suppliers, while increasing their own. The worst situation is one in which your suppliers have substantial market power and you have none. Your profit margins will not look very good.

The Impact of Market Structure on Markups

Analyses of the impact of market structure on markups are not routine, because they require information on both prices and costs, which are typically closely guarded by managers. There are a few healthcare studies, however, such as the one of nursing homes that found higher markups in areas in which there was greater market concentration (Nyman 1994). A market with a high degree of concentration either has relatively few competitors or has a few dominant firms. Economists often use the Hirschman-Herfindahl Index (HHI) to measure market concentration.

The HHI equals the sum of the squared market shares of the competitors in a market. As a result, the HHI gets larger as the number of firms gets smaller or as the market shares of the largest firms get larger. For example, a market with five firms, each of which claimed 20 percent of the market, would have an HHI of 2,000. In contrast, a market with five firms, four of which each claimed 15 percent of the market and one claimed 40 percent, would have an HHI of 2,500.

The study found that a one percent increase in the HHI was associated with a 0.13–0.15 percent increase in prices. This might not seem like much, but it implies that prices would be 3 or 4 percent higher in a market with an HHI of 2,500 than in a market with an HHI of 2,000. This sort of difference in markups should have a major impact on profits.

14.6 Market Power and Profits

Market power does not guarantee profits. The firm with market power will set price well above marginal cost, but may not earn an adequate return on equity. Earning a less inadequate return on equity than would be possible without market power is not much consolation. However, firms with market power can use strategies to boost profits that firms without market power cannot.

Three competitive strategies are common among firms with market power: price discrimination, product differentiation, and collusion. Price discrimination was discussed in Chapter 10; therefore, in this chapter we will focus on collusion and product differentiation.

14.6.1 Collusion

Collusion, or inspiring to limit competition, has a long history in medicine. As in other industries, the temptation to avoid the rigors of market competition can be beguiling, especially in healthcare. Collusion is quite profitable because demand is so much less elastic for the profession than for each individual participant. For example, if the price elasticity of demand for physicians' services is about -0.20 and the price elasticity of demand for an individual physician's services is about -3.00, each individual physician will perceive that she can increase her income by cutting prices, yet raising prices will increase the income of the profession as a whole.

Figure 14.2 shows how a 10 percent price increase would change total revenue for organizations facing different elasticities. (The change in total revenue due to price cut equals the percentage change in price plus the percentage change in quantity plus the percentage change in price times the percentage change in quantity.) For the profession as a whole, raising prices will increase revenues because demand is inelastic. For each individual professional, raising prices seems that it will reduce revenues, because demand is elastic as long as other professionals do not change their prices. Of course, others are likely to respond to price cuts by cutting prices themselves, so revenues are likely to climb far less than a naive analysis would suggest.

The implication of Figure 14.2 is that physicians as a group would increase their incomes if they refused to give discounts to managed care organizations. What is good for the profession, however, is not what is good for its individual members. Every individual physician would be tempted to decry managed-care

Price increase	Elasticity	Quantity change	Revenue change
10.0%	−0.1	−1.0%	8.9%
10.0%	−0.2	−2.0%	7.8%
10.0%	−0.3	−3.0%	6.7%
10.0%	−3.0	−30.0%	−23.0%
10.0%	−3.5	−35.0%	−28.5%
10.0%	−4.0	−40.0%	−34.0%

discounts, but make private deals with HMOs once the medical society meeting had concluded. From the perspective of the profession, what is needed is a way of penalizing defectors.

In the 1930s, Oregon physicians did just this. Faced with an oversupply of physicians, excess capacity in the state's hospitals, and widespread concern about the costs of healthcare, insurance companies in Oregon attempted to restrict use of physicians' services. Medical societies in Oregon responded by threatening to expel physicians who participated in these insurance plans. Because membership in a county medical society was usually required for a physician to have hospital privileges, this was a serious threat. This threat and the ultimate refusal of physicians to deal with insurance companies led the insurers to abandon efforts to restrict use of physicians' services (Starr 1982).

In most industries these steps would be recognized as illegal, anti-competitive activities. Until the 1970s, however, many observers believed that the antitrust laws did not apply to the medical profession. But a 1982 Supreme Court decision signaled that healthcare providers would be subject to antitrust laws. Since then the Federal Trade Commission has sued to prevent boycotts of insurers, efforts to deny hospital privileges to participants in managed-care plans, and attempts to restrict advertising. In short, healthcare professionals and healthcare organizations are to be treated no differently than others.

The benefits of collusion remain clear. By restricting competition, firms can reduce the price elasticity of demand and increase markups. Collusion only increases profits, however, until it is detected.

14.7 Product Differentiation and Advertising

Product differentiation takes two forms: attribute-based and information-based. In the first, customers recognize that two products have different attributes, even though they are fairly close substitutes. With this sort of **attribute-based** differentiation, customers may not respond to small price differences. In **information-based** product differentiation, customers have incomplete information about how well products suit their needs. Information is expensive to gather and verify, so customers are reluctant to switch products once they have identified one that is acceptable. Both of these forms of product differentiation reduce the price elasticity of demand for a product and create market power (Caves and Williamson 1985).

Both attribute-based and information-based product differentiation are prevalent in healthcare. For example, a board-certified pediatrician who practices on the west side of town very clearly provides a service that is different from a board-certified pediatrician who practices on the east side of town. If the two practices were closer, more customers would view them as equivalent. Alternatively, armed only with a general sense that the technical skills, interpersonal skills, and prices of surgeons can vary significantly, a potential customer who has found an acceptable surgeon is not likely to switch just because a neighbor reports that she was charged a lower fee for the same procedure. Of course, the customer might be more likely to switch if complication rates, patient satisfaction scores, and prices for both surgeons were posted on the Internet, so she could easily compare them.

The role of information differs sharply for attribute-based and information-based product differentiation. Extensive advertising makes sense for products with different attributes that matter to consumers. The more clearly that customers see the differences, the less elastic demand will be and the higher markups can be for "better" products. In contrast, restrictions on advertising (and even restrictions on disclosure of information) make sense when there is information-based product differentiation. The harder it is for customers to see that products do not differ in ways that matter to them, the less elastic demand will be and the higher markups can be.

The coexistence of attribute-based and information-based product differentiation in healthcare leads to some confusing advertising patterns. Attribute-based product differentiation almost demands advertising. Getting information about product differences into the hands of customers is an integral part of this type of product differentiation. For example, pharmaceutical manufacturers have launched extensive direct-to-consumer advertising campaigns. On the other hand, better customer information tends to erode the market power created by information-based product differentiation. Where this is common, as it is in much of healthcare, there is a temptation to try to restrict advertising. As you might suspect, the most successful limits have been based in state law, as private restrictions on advertising are usually illegal.

Despite these divergent incentives, advertising has a long history in healthcare, and it has increased in recent years. One reason, of course, has been the growing body of court rulings that make it clear that professional societies cannot limit advertising. It appears however, that advertising has also increased in some sectors, such as inpatient care, where advertising has long been legal. The real driving force seems to be increasing competition for patients.

The nature of healthcare products and the nature of healthcare markets should combine to make advertising quite common. To begin with, most healthcare firms have both market power and competition to some degree. It is in markets such as these that advertising is most common. Advertising helps differentiate one product from another, so it increases margins. In monopoly markets (e.g., the only hospital in an isolated town), such product differentiation is not useful. The provider already has high margins, and advertising is unlikely to increase them. In markets with a great many providers (e.g., retailers of over-the-counter pain medications), margins may be low, but it will be difficult to differentiate one seller from another and advertising expenditures will be unlikely to increase revenues.

In addition, it is difficult to assess the quality and general suitability of most healthcare goods and services before using them. Because of this, advertising can perform a useful service. Advertising can give consumers information that they would have difficulty getting otherwise. There is no real contradiction here. If consumers gained no information from advertising, they would probably ignore it. Having information about a product differentiates it from products about which one does not have information. Of course, those who offer exceptional values also need to advertise to ensure that consumers are aware of their low prices or high quality. Studies of advertising in healthcare generally find that banning advertising results in higher prices.

The economic logic behind advertising and innovating is quite simple: continue to do more as long as the increase in revenue is greater than the increase in cost. Stop when marginal revenue from advertising or product differentiation just equals the marginal costs. This differs from the standard rule only in that the marginal costs will include the cost of producing the good or service and the cost of differentiation (advertising or innovating). Figure 14.3 shows the calculations that organizations need to consider. As long as the incremental costs of production and advertising are less than the incremental revenue that results, increasing advertising will increase profits. What must be stressed is that managers need to take into account both advertising and production costs. Advertising only makes sense for products with significant margins.

The profit-maximizing amount of advertising depends on consumers' responses to both advertising and prices. The profit-maximizing rule is that advertising costs (measured as a percentage of sales) should equal $-\alpha/\varepsilon$. This rule of thumb predicts that profits will be maximized when an organization's advertising to sales ratio equals -1 multiplied by the ratio of the advertising elasticity of demand $[-\alpha]$ to the price elasticity of demand $[\varepsilon]$. As you might expect, the advertising elasticity of demand is the percentage increase in the quantity demanded when advertising expenses increase by one percent. Obviously, if advertising does not

FIGURE 14.3
Advertising and
Profits

| Incremental revenue | Incremental Cost | | Profits |
	of production	of advertising	
			$100,000
$50,000	$30,000	$10,000	$110,000
$50,000	$30,000	$22,000	$108,000

increase sales it is not worth doing. This rule also makes it clear that firms with less elastic demand will find it desirable to spend more on advertising. This rule implies that a firm with an advertising elasticity of demand of 0.1 should spend 2.5 percent of its revenues on advertising if its price elasticity of demand is -4.00, but another firm with $\alpha = 0.1$ should spend 5 percent of revenues on advertising if its price elasticity of demand is -2.00.

Product differentiation (whether through innovation or advertising) is a process, not an outcome. Differentiation, although potentially profitable, tends to erode. Product differentiation can be clear cut (e.g., an open MRI); less distinguishable (e.g., "Featuring patient-centered care"); barely noticeable (e.g., "Meals that don't taste like hospital food"); emotional (e.g., "Doctors who care"); or frivolous (e.g., stripes in tooth gel). In all of these instances, however, successful differentiation asks to be copied and generally is, thus necessitating ceaseless efforts to differentiate products.

Outside observers tend to think that product differentiation must be very difficult. It is not, but maintaining it is.

14.8 Conclusion

Most healthcare firms have some market power. Market power allows higher markups and can result in higher profits. As a result, firms unceasingly try to acquire market power or, if they have it, to defend it. The best way to acquire or defend market power is via regulation. Competitors find it more difficult to erode market power that has been gained by action of governments.

Organizations can also take steps to gain market power without government action. Common strategies include preemption, limit pricing, and innovation, all of which are designed to discourage potential entrants. Mergers can also result in market power, as can collusion with rivals. Unlike other strategies for gaining market power, mergers and collusion often create legal problems. Mergers may result in public or private anti-trust lawsuits, as will collusion once it has been discovered.

Firms with market power can compete in a variety of ways. Where feasible, firms seek to gain market power via product differentiation and advertising. This makes managers' roles more challenging. Of course, the profit potential of market power creates an incentive to seek it, even without a guarantee of profits.

References

Bamezai, A., J. Zwanziger, G. A. Melnick, and J. M. Mann. 1999. "Price Competition and Hospital Cost Growth in the United States." *Health Economics* 8 (3): 233–43.

Caves, R. E. and P. J. Williamson. 1985. "What is Product Differentiation, Really?" *The Journal of Industrial Economics* 34 (2)" 113–32.

Dranove, D. 1998. "Economies of Scale in Non-Revenue Producing Cost Centers: Implications for Hospital Mergers." *Journal of Health Economics* 17 (1): 69–83.

Keeler, E. B., G. Melnick, and J. Zwanziger. 1999. "The Changing Effects of Competition on Non-Profit and For-Profit Pricing Behavior." *Journal of Health Economics* 18 (1): 69–86.

Lee, R. H., and J. Hadley. 1981. "Physicians' Fees and Public Medical Care." *Health Services Research* 16 (2): 185–203.

McCarthy, T R. 1985. "The Competitive Nature of the Primary-Care Physician Services Market." *Journal of Health Economics* 4 (2): 93–117.

Nyman, J. A. 1994. "The Effects of Market Concentration and Excess Demand on the Price of Nursing Home Care." *Journal of Industrial Economics* 42 (2): 193–204.

Porter, M. E. 1985. *Competitive Advantage*. New York: Free Press.

Starr, P. 1982. *The Social Transformation of American Medicine*. New York: Basic, 205.

STRATEGIC BEHAVIOR

Key Concepts

- Strategic thinking is vital for most healthcare managers.
- Strategic thinking is essential in negotiating contracts.
- Clearly understanding your best option without a deal is a key to successful negotiation.
- Strategic thinking is essential in responding to initiatives by large rivals.
- Knowing your options and your rivals' options is an essential part of strategic thinking.
- A firm should pursue a dominant strategy no matter what its rival does.
- In a **Nash equilibrium** none of the players want to change what they are doing, given what the others are doing.
- Players can alter the outcomes of games by making credible threats or commitments.

15.1 Introduction

Strategic thinking is vital for most healthcare managers. In all types of markets, managers routinely negotiate contracts with other companies. Successful leadership in some markets demands skillful responses to the strategies of rivals. In hospital, nursing home, home health, insurance, and other healthcare markets, the quest for market power and economies of scale leads to an oligopolistic market (one with only a few competitors). In such a market, managers must ask, "If my rivals act effectively to realize their goals, how should I incorporate their likely behavior into my decision making?"

The answer to this question will not be simple. Indeed, **game theory** (which is the study of these situations) makes it clear that even simple strategy problems can have complex solutions. Sometimes formal analysis will be of no help. But in other cases, your best response to your rivals' strategies will be clear, and in some cases you will be able to influence what your rivals do.

Competing against a well-organized, aggressive rival is difficult, challenging a great many healthcare managers. In any market with only a few players, the competitors must track what the others are doing. Not responding to the initiatives of rivals can be damaging, especially in markets where growth is slow.

15.2 Bargaining

Game theory recognizes two types of games. In **cooperative games** the players can negotiate binding contracts. Here, managers need to understand the bargaining process that leads to efficient contracts, and when a contract will not be binding. Players in **noncooperative games** cannot negotiate binding contracts, but must "play" against one another. Noncooperative games, as you might suspect, resemble games like checkers, poker, and backgammon. Each player acts to further his or her own interest, and the more skillful player wins. Market competition differs from checkers, poker, and backgammon in that the resources available to the players can be quite different. "Winning" against a rival with more resources and lower costs may involve identifying a market niche in which your rival's strengths are negated.

15.2.1 Cooperative Games

Bargaining is the hallmark of cooperative games. Perhaps the most important aspect of bargaining is understanding the worst deal that both you and the other side will accept. Failure to agree is always a possibility in bargaining, and both sides need to gain from the bargain. This is true in both the short and long run. Parties seldom agree to terms that are worse than "no deal," and research confirms that "playing fair" is important. Negotiators may not agree to deals that they regard as unfair, even if the deal is better than their "no deal" option. Most negotiators will interact over and over, and even when this is not true, a bargainer's reputation generally becomes common knowledge. Unless it is advantageous to develop a reputation as a "crazy" or difficult person to do business with, a reputation for reliability and honesty will make bargaining easier and more rewarding. Using a partner's inexperience or lack of information to take advantage of him is a bad idea. Good managers should treasure their reputations, realizing that an opponent's belief in their good faith is their most valuable asset, and never let their honesty come into question (Shister 1997).

One of the hallmarks of strategic thinking is a recognition that some short-term gains will result in long-term losses. The gains from bargaining need not be distributed equally. One party is often in a much stronger position than the other, or may have better options or less to lose if the negotiations break down. The art of negotiation is to press this advantage just far enough, but no further. Creating an enemy in the process of crafting an agreement is dangerous. On the other hand, a party in a weak negotiating position should not expect to share equally in the rewards of an agreement.

Most of what managers do involves negotiation. Negotiation plays an important role in contracts with suppliers, sales to customers, agreements with partners, deals with peers, and arrangements with subordinates. Yet many managers do not think systematically about these negotiations (Ertel 1999). In particular, many assume that negotiation always represents a zero-sum game, in which one party's gains equal another party's losses.

This is not always true. Some negotiations can result in gains for all the parties. Most business relationships are not short term, so a natural question to ask is whether a negotiation strengthened or weakened the relationship between the parties. From this flow three questions about how the bargaining process affected the relationship. Did the negotiation allow the parties to converse about problem solving? Did the negotiation explore innovations that might let all parties win? Did the negotiation advance the interests of all the parties? Of course, if these sorts of criteria are to matter, they must be the criteria that drive the incentives—bonuses, commissions, promotions, or non-financial rewards—that negotiators face. Otherwise, these criteria will be just rhetoric, and no one will pay any attention to them.

Negotiators can also seek to change the game when they propose alternatives. For example, a supply firm that allows just-in-time ordering by unit staff reduces inventory and acquisition costs for its customer. At the same time, just-in-time ordering makes other vendors less competitive, so the bargaining process should put less pressure on margins.

Bargaining needs to result in a contract that benefits both parties. If not, it makes no sense to sign. By the same token, unless it is in the interests of your partner to carry out the agreement that you have crafted, it is a bad agreement. Contracts need to be enforceable, and enforceable at low cost. An agreement that forces your partner to do something that he does not want to do is likely to fail. Turning to the courts to enforce a contract or keeping the bond that your partner has posted generally means that you have not gotten what you wanted. An enforceable contract is one that both partners want to live up to. An important part of the art of negotiating is the ability to write a contract that neither party wants to breach.

The Importance of Bargaining in Healthcare

Bargaining has become more important in healthcare than ever before. One attribute that distinguishes managed care plans from traditional insurers is a reliance on negotiated prices. Managed care plans typically bargain with providers about prices, and the expansion of pharmaceutical insurance means that pharmacies must bargain as well. Pharmacy trade associations have argued that managed care plans have failed to bargain in good faith, offering "take it or leave it" deals that unsophisticated pharmacists accept. Even though this is an accurate description of the contracting mechanism, in that face-to-face bargaining sessions are uncommon, it appears to misrepresent the amount of bargaining power that pharmacists have. Indeed, the Federal Trade Commission has objected to some recent pharmacy mergers, fearing that market concentration would drive up prices. In addition, an analysis of managed care contracts with pharmacies suggests that, although there are seldom formal negotiating sessions, pharmacies get better prices when their bargaining position is stronger (Brooks et al. 1999).

Managed care pharmacy contracts usually specify a discount from list price (called Average Wholesale Price) plus a dispensing fee. The terms of these contracts appear to reflect the relative bargaining positions of pharmacies and managed care organizations. Factors that improve the bargaining position of pharmacies result in higher prices; those that improve the bargaining position of managed care firms result in lower prices. For example, prices tend to be higher when there are few pharmacies in an area or when ownership is highly concentrated. Prices tend to be lower when the insurer has a larger share of the local market. Independent pharmacies tend to get paid a bit more than chain pharmacies, probably reflecting their higher costs. In short, even though bargaining with managed care firms largely consists of pharmacies accepting or rejecting the firms' offers, this process has results much like those of face-to-face bargaining.

15.2.2 *Noncooperative Games*

Cooperative games are complex, but noncooperative games are far more complex, because neither the rules nor the agreements are written down. In competing in oligopoly markets, managers need to focus on five key issues:

1. Know your options.
2. Know your rival's options.
3. Understand your rival's point of view.
4. Forecast your rival's responses to your initiatives or changes in the market.
5. Influence your rival's responses.

All of these are important, but by far the most important is understanding your reasonable options. Only by luck will a manager who has not identified the options open to her succeed. Knowing what can be done and what cannot be done is essential. If you have not thought of a strategy, you will not pursue it. If you have not seen that a strategy is impractical, you may waste time trying to implement it. The worst mistakes usually involve ignoring an important option. Ignoring one of your rival's options can also be disastrous.

An Example of Preemptive Strategy

In 1988 both Baptist Memorial Hospital and Methodist Hospitals of Memphis submitted Certificate of Need applications to the Tennessee Health Facilities Commission to authorize the purchase of positron emission tomography [PET] equipment. The Commission approved both applications, yet neither hospital actually purchased the equipment. Three years later, the two hospitals signed a joint venture agreement to provide PET. To date, the joint venture has not purchased the PET equipment. The explanation for this odd sequence of events lies in strategic considerations, according to a recent analysis (Weingarten 1999).

Interviews with senior managers confirmed that both Baptist and Methodist proceeded with PET Certificate of Need applications mainly to preempt each other. Neither had much confidence that PET would be very profitable. Many insurers did not cover it, considering it experimental, and demand forecasts for PET were nebulous. Even more importantly, neither manager was responding to concerted advocacy by physicians. Given PET's high cost, delay seemed the logical decision, yet neither wanted the other hospital to be the recipient of the sole Certificate of Need.

When the Commission unexpectedly granted both Certificates of Need, a new preemption strategy was needed. The joint venture was a creative way to insure that neither would be left without PET, if it should become a standard part of tertiary radiology. The joint venture prevented either of the partners from proceeding independently, and neither was concerned about other hospitals, as there were no plausible alternative PET providers in Memphis. The joint venture also represented an option on the technology. If equipment prices fell and PET became more widely accepted, the joint venture would allow the hospitals to proceed. The joint venture also converted the noncooperative preemption game in which both were likely to suffer losses into a cooperative game in which neither stood to lose.

15.3 Dominant Strategies

Is there a dominant strategy? Managers must ask several questions to answer this: Will my best strategy be the same no matter what my rival does? Will my rival's best strategy be the same no matter what I do? In Figure 15.1, Bethany has a dominant strategy. No matter what Avalon does, Bethany should accept the PPO contract. (Avalon's choices are listed along the left side of the table, and Bethany's choices are listed along the top of the table.) If Avalon joins the PPO, Bethany will earn $200 if it joins and only $100 if it does not. If Avalon does not join the PPO, Bethany will earn $450 if it joins and only $400 if it does not. This gives the managers of Avalon an important insight. Their planning has become much simpler. Bethany should join the PPO no matter what, so Avalon's managers need only choose the best strategy, given this fact. In this instance, Avalon should also join the PPO. Note, however, that Avalon does not have a dominant strategy. Avalon's best strategy is to join when Bethany does and to refuse to join when Bethany does not. (To understand a game, consider each option open to a player and then identify its rival's best response. Then identify the player's best response for each of the rival's options.)

Figure 15.1 is a payoff matrix. A payoff matrix tries to write down each player's possible strategies and forecast the gain (or payoff) that each will realize. For example, Figure 15.1 predicts that Avalon will get a payoff of 400 and Bethany will get a payoff of 200 if both accept the PPO contract. Obviously the payoff forecasts are largely conjectures, but they need not be precise to be helpful. For

FIGURE 15.1
Accepting a PPO
Contract as a
Dominant Strategy

Avalon	Bethany	
	Accept PPO contract	Refuse PPO contract
Accept PPO contract	$Y_A = 400, Y_B = 200$	$Y_A = 600, Y_B = 100$
Refuse PPO contract	$Y_A = 100, Y_B = 450$	$Y_A = 700, Y_B = 400$

example, the results in Figure 15.1 reflect three simple rules. First, joining the PPO reduces prices and profits, with two significant exceptions. Second, a firm whose rival has joined the PPO can increase market share and profits by also joining. Third, Bethany has enough excess capacity so that its profits will rise if it joins the PPO and Avalon does not. Any set of payoffs that follow these rules would force the same conclusions as Figure 15.1. The fact that the forecasts are "guestimates" does not reduce the value of trying to lay out a payoff matrix. The real value of this process comes from thinking systematically about your options, your opponents' options, and the resulting payoffs. Simply writing down your options and your rival's options can clarify the situation quite a bit. It also makes it easier for others to add options that you haven't considered or critique your assumptions about payoffs. It may then be obvious what your rival is going to do (whether you like it or not) or what you should do.

The game in 15.1 has an equilibrium outcome. Once both have accepted the PPO contract, neither will want to defect. Bethany's income would fall if it dropped out of the PPO, as would Avalon's. Neither wants to change what it is doing, given what the other is doing. This type of strategic equilibrium is called a **Nash equilibrium**, after the mathematician who developed it in the 1950s. This equilibrium will persist even though both firms would prefer an environment in which neither of them accepted the PPO contract. Both of them refusing to sign is not an equilibrium, however. Bethany has an incentive to defect, since its income is highest when it accepts the PPO contract and Avalon does not. So, both firms refusing to contract with the PPO is not a Nash equilibrium.

Games of this type are often called "prisoner's dilemma" games, in that the outcome that both parties prefer is not an equilibrium. The name comes from a game in which prisoners are questioned separately. Neither will be convicted if the other does not confess, but the promise of a reduced sentence induces both to confess, so both draw long sentences. Managers do not want to play a prisoner's dilemma game. Below we will look at ways that the players can avoid such games.

Small changes in market conditions can lead to very different outcomes. In Figure 15.2, only one number has changed from Figure 15.1. Bethany's income is forecast to be only $350 instead of $450 when it accepts the PPO contract and Avalon does not. This change means that accepting the PPO contract is no longer a dominant strategy for Bethany. It also means that this game has two possible Nash equilibria. One continues to be that both accept. The other is that both

Avalon	Bethany	
	Accept PPO contract	Refuse PPO contract
Accept PPO contract	$Y_A = 400, Y_B = 200$	$Y_A = 600, Y_B = 100$
Refuse PPO contract	$Y_A = 100, Y_B = 350$	$Y_A = 700, Y_B = 400$

FIGURE 15.2
A Game With No
Dominant Strategy

refuse. Verify that neither would want to defect from either of these equilibria. Neither Bethany nor Avalon does better by defecting when the equilibrium is Accept-Accept or Refuse-Refuse.

This example illustrates two important features of strategic behavior. First, contests can have many different outcomes, and managers may prefer some of those outcomes much more than others. Second, by changing payoffs, managers can change the outcomes of games.

15.4 Repeated Games

Most business relationships are long-term. This can fundamentally change the winning strategy. As the old saying notes, "Fool me once, your fault. Fool me twice, my fault." When players (organizations or individuals) interact repeatedly, the range of sensible strategies expands. Threats of future retribution may provide an escape route from aggressive price competition, or a player's reputation may costlessly deter entry by rivals.

Figure 15.3 describes the payoffs for a game involving entry. Universal already provides managed behavioral health services in a local market. It is the only significant player and realizes handsome profits. The managers of Global must assess whether they should enter this market. If they believe, based on its behavior in other markets, that Universal will ultimately be a sensible rival, Global will enter the market and its profits will be 200, because Universal will not start a price war if Global enters.

Suppose, on the other hand, that Universal recognizes that the only way for it to enjoy continued high profits is to develop a reputation as an "irrational" competitor. It makes it clear that it evaluates its regional managers primarily in terms of market share and only secondarily in terms of profits. A manager who delivers high profits gets bonuses, but a manager who loses market share gets

Universal	Global	
	Enter market	Does not enter market
Share the market	$Y_U = 200, Y_G = 200$	$Y_U = 600, Y_G = 0$
Start a price war	$Y_U = -5, Y_G = -5$	$Y_U = 400, Y_G = 0$

FIGURE 15.3
Universal Is a
Rational Incumbent

FIGURE 15.4
Universal Is an
Irrational
Incumbent

Universal	Global	
	Enter market	Does not enter market
Share the market	$Y_U = -20, Y_G = 200$	$Y_U = 600, Y_G = 0$
Start a price war	$Y_U = -5, Y_G = -5$	$Y_U = 400, Y_G = 0$

fired. So Global or any other competitor must recognize that regional managers will defend market share with a passion. As Figure 15.4 makes clear, it is sensible for Universal's managers to start a price war, even though that will hurt Universal's profits and their bonuses. Their payoff for sensible post-entry behavior is negative because of this policy. Armed with the knowledge that Universal is an irrational competitor, Global will not want to enter its market. As a result, the irrational competitor can forestall entry, because potential rivals do not want to compete with an irrational adversary. Of course, Universal may have to launch a vigorous price war when a rival enters the market, to emphasize that they are serious.

Both Universal and its rivals understand that the most profitable outcome of all will be if it appears to be irrational but really is not. The appearance of irrationality will keep most rivals out, but the actual price war that follows entry is quite costly (plus Universal hates to fire competent managers just because they have lost some market share).

Having a reputation is one way that repeated play changes the game. Repeated play also lets participants make credible threats and commitments. If a player can make a credible threat or commitment, she can change the equilibrium.

15.5 Credible Threats and Commitments

A credible threat is a strategy that punishes your opponent and represents your best response to your rival's action. In Figure 15.5 Avalon makes an *incredible* threat to join an HMO if Bethany enters the market. The threat is not credible because, given that Bethany has entered the market, Avalon's best response is to refuse to join the HMO. Therefore, even though Avalon has the capacity to punish Bethany for entering the market, Bethany will ignore the threat. Ignoring incredible threats is the winning course of action in bargaining or strategy.

FIGURE 15.5
Avalon's Threat to
Join the HMO if
Bethany Enters the
Market Is Not
Credible

Avalon	Bethany	
	Enter market	Does not enter market
Join HMO	$Y_A = 300, Y_B = -10$	$Y_A = 600, Y_B = 0$
Do not join HMO	$Y_A = 400, Y_B = 300$	$Y_A = 700, Y_B = 0$

Avalon	Bethany	
	Enter market	Does not enter market
Join HMO	$Y_A = 200, Y_B = -10$	$Y_A = 600, Y_B = 0$
Do not join HMO	$Y_A = 100, Y_B = 300$	$Y_A = 600, Y_B = 0$

FIGURE 15.6
Avalon's Threat to Join HMO if Bethany Enters the Market Is Credible

Avalon	Bethany	
	Accept PPO contract	Refuse PPO contract
Accept PPO contract	$Y_A = 400, Y_B = 200$	$Y_A = 600, Y_B = 100$
Refuse PPO contract	$Y_A = 100, Y_B = 450$	$Y_A = 700, Y_B = 400$

FIGURE 15.7
Accepting a PPO Contract as a Dominant Strategy

Avalon can force Bethany to respect its threat by changing its circumstances. For example, Avalon could build enough capacity to make joining the HMO its best strategy if Bethany enters the market. In Figure 15.6, Bethany would be wise to respect Avalon's threat, because if Bethany enters the market, Avalon really has no choice but to join the HMO. That being the case, Bethany will not want to enter.

Recall that, in our initial example of a noncooperative game, accepting a PPO contract was a dominant strategy for Bethany. (Figure 15.7 reproduces that example.) Bethany has an incentive to defect from the Refuse-Refuse outcome, and neither player has an incentive to defect from the Accept-Accept outcome.

With only two of them replaying this game over and over, Avalon and Bethany might be able to monitor cheating and successfully avoid accepting the PPO contract (or sign, but offer little or no discount). A simple tit-for-tat strategy might well work. In such a strategy, Bethany would make it clear that it planned to refuse the PPO contract, but if Avalon accepted it would join as well, and profits would fall for both. As long as both parties expect to play indefinitely and do not expect entry by other organizations, this simple strategy might well support a Refuse-Refuse equilibrium. Neither would want to defect because of the long-term consequences.

If there were more players, however, a player would eventually offer discounts to gain market share. Or, if entry were possible, someone would eventually conclude that the system of tacit cooperation was about to collapse and would defect. With large numbers of rivals or with easy entry, tacit cooperation is almost sure to break down. When it does, price competition becomes the norm and margins get squeezed. Of course, individual organizations can still try to differentiate their products and gain higher markups.

15.6 Conclusion

The main feature that sets markets with only a few participants apart from other markets is that firms recognize their mutual interdependence. That is, the best strategy for one player depends on the strategy chosen by the others. Each needs to be concerned with what its rivals are doing, watching carefully to predict what they will do. Because of this interdependence, oligopolists face a complex decision-making process. Each must determine its best response to its opponents' strategies and try to deduce what it should do. As you can imagine, this can get very complex very quickly.

Equilibrium in an oligopoly market occurs when no participant wants to change its strategy, given what the other participants are doing. In other words, it is in each firm's self-interest to continue producing the equilibrium quantity of goods, or to continue setting prices at the equilibrium level.

The game of business competition can be quite complex; however, remembering the five key issues can help you bargain and compete successfully:

1. Know your options.
2. Know your rival's options.
3. Understand your rival's point of view.
4. Forecast your rival's responses to changed circumstances.
5. Influence your rival's responses via credible threats.

References

Brooks, J. M., W. Doucette, and B. Sorofman. 1999. "Factors Affecting Bargaining Outcomes Between Pharmacies and Insurers." *Health Services Research* 34 (1) Part II: 439–51.

Ertel, D. 1999. "Turning Negotiation into a Corporate Capability." *Harvard Business Review* 77 (3): 55–70.

Shister, N. 1997. *10 Minute Guide to Negotiating.* New York: Macmillan Spectrum, 13.

Weingarten, J. P., Jr. 1999. "Cooperative Ventures in a Competitive Environment: The Influence of Regulation on Management Decisions." *Journal of Healthcare Management* 44 (4): 282–300.

GLOSSARY

Adverse selection. Occurs when individuals with a greater-than-average need for medical care enroll in a healthcare plan in a larger proportion than they exist in the general population.

Agency. An arrangement in which one person (the agent) takes actions on behalf of another (the principal).

Asymmetric information. Asymmetric information is present when one party to a transaction has better information about it than another.

Attribute-based product differentiation. In this type of product differentiation, consumers recognize that different products have different attributes, even though they are fairly close substitutes.

Average cost. Average cost = total cost / total output.

Benefits. Benefits measure the value of goods or services, most commonly in terms of what individuals would willingly exchange for them.

Capitation. Capitation consists of a flat payment to a provider per person cared for. The provider assumes the risk that the payment will cover the cost of the patient's care.

Carve out. If a capitation contract makes another organization responsible for a type of service, that service has been carved out of the capitation contract.

Case-based payment. Case-based payment consists of a single payment for an episode of care. The payment does not change if fewer services or more services are provided.

Complement. A complement is a product used in conjunction with another product.

Cooperative game. In a cooperative game the players can negotiate binding contracts.

Copayment. A copayment is a fee that the patient must pay in addition to the amount paid by insurance.

Cost. Cost is the value of a resource in its next-best use.

Cost sharing. Cost sharing is the general term for direct payments to providers by insurance beneficiaries. Deductibles, copayments, and coinsurance are forms of cost sharing.

Cost shifting. In this hypothesis, it is believed that price reductions for some will increase costs for others.

Cross-price elasticity. The percentage change in the quantity demanded that is associated with a one percent change in the price of a substitute or complement.

Credible threat. A credible threat punishes a rival and is the best response to the rival's action.

Demand. Demand describes the amounts of a good or service that will be purchased at different prices when all other factors are held constant.

Demand curve. A demand curve describes how much consumers are willing to buy of a specific product at different prices.

Demand shift. A demand shift occurs when a factor other than price (e.g., consumer incomes) changes.

Diagnosis-related groups. Diagnosis-related groups (DRGs) are the case groups that underlie Medicare's case-based payment system to hospitals.

Discounting. Discounting adjusts the value of future costs and benefits to reflect the willingness of consumers to trade current consumption for future consumption. Usually future values are discounted by $1/(1 + r)^n$, with r being the discount rate and n the number of periods in the future that the cost or benefit will be realized.

Dominant strategy. A dominant strategy is advantageous to pursue no matter what rivals do.

Economies of scale. Economies of scale mean that large organizations have lower costs.

Economies of scope. Economies of scope mean that multiproduct organizations have lower production costs.

Efficiency. An efficient organization produces the most valuable output possible, given its inputs. Viewed differently, an efficient organization uses the least expensive inputs possible, given the quality and quantity of output that it produces.

Elastic. If the quantity of a product that is demanded falls by more than one percent when the price of the product rises by one percent, demand is elastic. This term is usually applied only to price elasticities of demand.

Elasticity. An elasticity is the percent change in a dependent variable associated with a one percent change in an independent variable.

Equilibrium price. At the equilibrium price the quantity demanded equals the quantity supplied. No shortage or surplus exists.

Equity. Equity is an organization's total assets minus outside claims on those assets.

Expected value. An expected value is an average that uses the probability of occurrence to weight possible outcomes.

Externality. An externality is a benefit or cost imposed on someone who is not a party to the transaction that causes it.

Factor of production. A factor of production is another name for an input.

Fee-for-Service (FFS). A fee-for-service insurance plan pays providers based on their charges for services.

Fixed costs. Fixed costs are costs that do not vary with output.

Gain sharing. Gain sharing is a general strategy for rewarding those who contribute to the success of an organization. Profit sharing is one form of gain sharing. Rewards can be based on other criteria as well.

Game theory. Game theory is the analysis of strategies to anticipate your rivals' actions.

Gross domestic product (GDP). The gross domestic product is the value of final goods and services that have been produced using domestic inputs. Gross domestic product seeks to measure the national output.

Group model HMO. A group model HMO contracts with a physician group to provide services.

Health Care Financing Administration (HCFA). HCFA is the federal agency charged with managing Medicare and working with the states to manage Medicaid.

Health maintenance organization (HMO). A health maintenance organization is a firm that provides comprehensive healthcare benefits to enrollees in exchange for a premium. Originally, HMOs were distinct from other insurance firms because providers were not paid on a fee-for-service basis and because enrollees faced no cost-sharing requirements. These distinctions no longer hold.

Income elasticity of demand. The income elasticity of demand is the percentage change in the quantity demanded that is associated with a one percent increase in income.

Increase or decrease in demand. An increase or decrease in demand is a shift in the entire list of amounts of a product that will be purchased at different prices.

Incremental cost. Incremental cost equals the change in cost due to a change in output.

Inelastic. If the quantity of a product demanded falls by less than one percent when the price rises by one percent, demand is inelastic. This term is usually applied only to price elasticities of demand.

Infant mortality rate. The infant mortality rate is the number of infant deaths in a year divided by the number of live births.

Information-based product differentiation. In this type of product differentiation, consumers have incomplete information about how well products suit their needs, making it difficult to compare different products.

Input. An input is a good or service that is used in the production of another good or service.

Interest group model of regulation. This model argues that regulations may be seen as attempts to further the interests of affected groups, usually producer groups.

Life year. A life year is one additional year of life for an individual. A life year can also represent 1/nth of a year of life for n individuals.

Limit pricing. Setting prices low enough to discourage entry into a market is called limit pricing.

Managed care. Managed care is a loosely defined term that includes PPO and

HMO plans. In managed care, the insurance plan is interposed between the patient and the provider and ultimately decides what services will be rendered.

Marginal analysis. Marginal analysis entails assessing the effects of small changes in a decision variable (such as price or the volume of output) on outcomes (such as costs, profits, or the probability of recovery).

Marginal cost pricing. Marginal cost pricing uses information about marginal costs and the price elasticity of demand to set profit-maximizing prices.

Marginal or incremental cost. A marginal or incremental cost is the cost of producing an additional unit of output.

Marginal revenue. This is the change in total revenue associated with a change in output.

Market demand. Market demand is the sum of the demands of all consumers in a market.

Market system. A market system uses prices to ration goods and services.

Medicaid. Medicaid is the name given to a collection of state programs that meet standards set by the Health Care Financing Administration, but which are run by state agencies. Medicaid serves those with incomes low enough to qualify for their state's program.

Medicare. Medicare is an insurance program for the elderly and disabled that is run by the Health Care Financing Administration, a federal agency.

Medicare Part A. Medicare Part A covers inpatient hospital, skilled nursing, hospice, and home healthcare services.

Medicare Part B. Medicare Part B covers outpatient services and medical equipment.

Modeling. Modeling costs entails identifying the perspective involved, the resources used, and the opportunity costs of those resources.

Monopolist. A monopolist is a firm with no rivals.

Monopolistic competitor. A monopolistic competitor has multiple rivals, but their products are imperfect substitutes.

Moral hazard. The incentive to use additional care that having insurance creates is called moral hazard.

Multi-part pricing. Multi-part pricing has separate fees for "membership" and service use.

Nash equilibrium. In a Nash equilibrium none of the participants want to change strategies, given what the others are doing.

Noncooperative game. In a noncooperative game the players cannot negotiate binding contracts.

Non-durable good. A good that is expected to be used up or wear out in a short period of time is non-durable.

Normal rate of return. A normal rate of return is a profit rate that is just high enough to retain current factors of production in an industry or occupation and low enough not to attract new entrants. A normal rate of return will equal the opportunity cost of the factors.

Normative economics. Normative economics uses values to assess and identify options regarding ethical, value, and factual judgments, and to analyze what to do given a set of circumstances.

Objective probability. An objective probability is based on the frequency of occurrence.

Oligopoly. An oligopoly is a firm with only a few rivals or a firm with only a few large rivals.

Opportunism. Opportunism is when an agent has better (or asymmetrical) information about a transaction and uses it to take advantage of another party (or principal).

Opportunity cost. A resource's opportunity cost is its value in its next best use. The opportunity cost of a product consists of the goods and services that we cannot have because we have chosen to produce it.

Out-of-pocket. The amount of money that a consumer directly pays for a good or service is the out-of-pocket cost.

Output. An output is the good or service that emerges from a production process.

Positive economics. Positive economics describes the world, using analysis and evidence to answer questions about individuals, organizations, and societies.

Preemption. Preemption consists of building enough excess capacity in a market so that potential entrants are discouraged.

Price discrimination. Selling similar goods or services to different individuals at different prices is price discrimination.

Price elasticity of demand. The percentage change in the quantity demanded that is associated with a one percent change in the price of a product.

Principal. A principal is the organization or individual represented by an agent.

Production to order. In production to order, organizations set prices and then fill their customers' orders.

Production to stock. In production to stock, organizations produce output and then adjust prices to sell what they have produced.

Profit. Profits are the difference between total revenue and total cost.

Quantity demanded. The quantity demanded is the amount of a good or service that will be purchased at a specific price when all other factors are held constant.

Real value. Real values have been adjusted for the effects of inflation using a price index.

Resources. Resources include anything that is useful in production or consumption.

Risk averse. A risk-averse decision maker is willing to accept an option with a lower expected value if it has less variability.

Risk neutral. A risk-neutral decision maker chooses the option with the highest expected value.

Risk seeking. A risk-seeking decision maker is willing to accept an option with a lower expected value if it has more variability.

Salary. A salary is a payment per period of time, and not directly related to output.

Scarce resources. Scarce resources are resources with multiple uses.

Sensitivity analysis. A sensitivity analysis substitutes alternative plausible values in calculations.

Shift in demand. A shift in demand occurs when one of the factors (e.g., consumer incomes) other than the price of the product itself changes.

Shift in supply. A shift in supply occurs when one of the factors (e.g., an input price) other than price changes.

Societal perspective. A societal perspective takes account of all costs and benefits, no matter to whom they accrue.

Staff Model HMO. A staff model HMO directly employs staff physicians to provide services.

Subjective probability. A subjective probability is based on the perceptions of decision makers.

Substitute. A substitute is a product used in place of another product.

Sunk costs. A sunk cost is any cost that cannot be changed (such as the purchase price of equipment or what is spent to train employees to use the equipment).

Supply curve. A supply curve describes how much producers are willing to sell at different prices.

Supply shift. A supply shift occurs when one of the factors (e.g., an input price) other than price changes.

Tying. A price strategy that links the prices of multiple products together, to balance multiple prices and maximize profits.

Underwriting. Underwriting is the process of assessing the risks associated with an insurance policy and setting the premium accordingly.

Utilization review. Analysis of patterns of resource use is called utilization review.

Variable costs. Costs that can vary with sales or output.

INDEX

About the Author

Robert H. Lee, Ph.D. is an associate professor in the Department of Health Policy and Management of the School of Medicine of the University of Kansas. Before joining the University of Kansas he was at the University of North Carolina, the Health Policy Program of the Urban Institute, and the Brookings Institution. He has published more than 20 healthcare economics articles.

Dr. Lee received a B.A. degree from Williams College and a Ph.D. from Johns Hopkins University.

Dr. Lee is an active member of the Association of University Programs in Health Administration, the Association for Health Services Research, and the International Health Economics Association.